The Beauty Geek's Guide to Skin Care

THE BEAUTY GEEK'S GUIDE TO

Skin Care

1,000 Essential Definitions of
Common Product Ingredients

DEBORAH BURNES

ROCKRIDGE
PRESS

For general information on our other products and services or to obtain technical support, please contact our Customer Care Department within the United States at (866) 744-2665, or outside the United States at (510) 253-0500.

Rockridge Press publishes its books in a variety of electronic and print formats. Some content that appears in print may not be available in electronic books, and vice versa.

Interior Designer: Peatra Jariya
Cover Designers: Eric Pratt and Jami Spittler
Editor: Nana K. Twumasi
Production Editor: Erum Khan
Photography © Sharlotta/iStock, cover, p. 126; Sirocco/shutterstock, pp. ii, iv; aimy27feb/iStock, pp. vii, ix; forest_strider/iStock, p. x; OksanaKiian/iStock, p. 8; imagehub88/iStock, p. 10; WEKWEK/iStock, p. 18.
Illustrations © solar22/iStock, p. 2.
Author photo © Gerald Bybee

ISBN: Print 978-1-64152-359-2 | eBook 978-1-64152-360-8

I HAVE BEEN INSPIRED

and privileged to know and love so many young women. My two daughters, two goddaughters, and the many wonderful friends of my children and staff members have filled my heart with love and joy. It is in watching these young women find their voice, make conscious choices and contributions, question, learn, listen, and make their way through life that moves me. These amazing women are filled with insight and the desire to grow, learn, and change. I dedicate this book to all these beautiful women, who define what beauty truly means.

CONTENTS

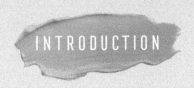

INTRODUCTION

ALTHOUGH I STARTED MY CAREER
working as a model in front of the camera, I decided to go to
cosmetology school to learn what the hair and makeup artists
were doing that made me look so fantastic. Instead, I fell deeply
and passionately in love with skin.

Skin is not only our largest organ; it is also literally the barrier between us and the world. It helps ward off illness and can even be a diagnosis tool for many ailments that first affect the skin. At first, I did not realize how deeply affected people are when struggling with issues such as severe acne, redness, or eczema, for example, but I have learned that the health of one's skin can also be a factor in one's mental health. When I was first able to transform a young woman's skin with my own acne-fighting products, her emotions were so profound I realized that working with skin is much more than skin-deep. This young woman, who had been embarrassed to be seen in public, who made herself into a social outcast, became more confident. She started going to school daily, and her depression lifted. She'd been so distraught about her appearance, and to see her change only solidified my passion for working with skin. It made me understand that working with people's skin makes it possible for them to see beyond their reflection in the mirror.

Early on in my career, I discovered I couldn't get the results I wanted from the products available on the market, so in 1997 I formulated Sumbody, one of the very first all-natural skin care brands. This was long before the onslaught of independent beauty and the popularity of being "all natural." I am a trained aesthetician and the cosmetic formulator behind Sumbody, for which I source each and every ingredient and manage the manufacturing of all our skin care products.

We've seen the momentum for eating healthy catapult to significant levels—health food grocery stores have become big chains, when before they used to be tucked-away treasures. Culturally, we are more aware of the hazards of eating fast foods, processed foods, and white sugar, and we are replacing them with fresh fruits and vegetables, whole grains, and beans. But what you may not know is that we absorb more toxins *through* our skin. If you're eating an organic apple but soaking in a tub of chemical soup, you'd be better off eating a conventionally grown apple and soaking in nontoxic ingredients. If you need evidence of how simple it is to absorb substances through our skin, consider nicotine patches, pain relief patches, and even birth control patches. Transdermal penetration is a fantastic vehicle for many things. Substances can penetrate on their own, but in the cosmetic industry we use "penetration enhancers" such as propylene glycol to help all the ingredients in a product get into your skin deeper than it might on its own.

Some years ago, I was the keynote speaker at the Society of Cosmetic Chemists. The topic was "What Is Natural?" Before I spoke, a group of chemists had debated this very topic, so when I gave my speech,

....

My goal is to make it simple for everyone to understand the options and decide what's best for their skin.

....

I said, "I couldn't have planned this debate any better to illustrate my point. If we as a group of cosmetic chemists cannot agree on what 'natural' means, how can we expect the public to understand and make choices in line with their personal beliefs? If we as an industry do not have better laws regarding what we can say on a label—such as 'all natural,' 'hypoallergenic,' and 'eco-friendly'—how can we expect the consumer to interpret a label? You shouldn't need to go back to chemistry class to understand what is in a product."

With this book, my goal is to make it simple for everyone to understand the options and decide what's best for their skin. I want to begin by making an important distinction: Not all things that are natural are good for you, and not everything that's synthetic is inherently toxic. Natural substances, like cyanide, for example, can be extremely harmful. Some synthetic substances, such as hyaluronic acid, are actually derived from natural sources. I believe it is necessary to change the conversation from "natural" versus "synthetic" to "healthy" versus "harmful."

As we discussed, skin is both your largest organ and a pathway for chemicals to enter your body. What you put on your skin is important. No one can decide for you, so I am presenting you with information to make informed choices about what you purchase and use. To keep things simple, I suggest that you primarily use products that include ingredients you can understand or easily identify, such as rose hip oil (page 105) and French green clay (page 57), instead of propylene glycol (page 101) and sodium laureth sulfate (page 111). Disregard what's on the front of a brand's label—it exists only to sell to you—and always flip the product around to read the ingredients list. Use this book as your source to make sure you're putting what's best for you on one of your most precious organs.

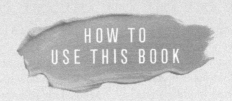

HOW TO USE THIS BOOK

I'VE SPENT MY CAREER EDUCATING PEOPLE
so they can make choices that align with their personal beliefs.
Even though I vehemently believe it's important for people to
understand the negative health effects of smoking cigarettes,
I would never impose my beliefs on someone else. What I can do
is give them information (the damaging effects of smoking)
that will allow them to make an educated choice.

The beauty industry has had backdoor access to our health without telling us what we need to know to make the choices that work for us. To that end, this book encompasses everything you need to understand your skin—how it works, what it needs to stay healthy, how to make choices aligned with your health goals, and tips and tricks of what to avoid/look for.

Having basic knowledge about skin and what it truly needs, along with guidelines for how to decipher the products you use, will arm you with the tools you need to make healthy and impactful choices in skin care. When you use the right products and understand how to care for your skin, you'll see your skin transform.

While the first two parts of this book talk about the what and how and why of skin, the bulk of the book is a comprehensive list of common cosmetic ingredients and terms. This is the backbone that will enable you

to choose products that will be effective and healthy. This book is meant to take the guesswork and confusion out of what's in a bottle. It puts the power in your hands. You'll learn where many ingredients fall on the "good for you/not good for you" scale, and with this information you'll be able to better assess whether a certain ingredient is appropriate for you.

Whether you're looking for the right ingredients to use in your DIY products, to understand what's in your current skin care routine, or as a go-to resource, this book will become an indispensable guide. It can also help you decide what you want to keep or eliminate from your existing routine. To address this specifically, I suggest taking all the products you and/or your family use and placing them in separate baskets or piles. I have been doing "green" make-overs with clients for years, and this is the first thing I do when I start working with a client. Even babies have their own piles of products! To do this on your own, eliminate all products that you haven't used in two months or more. Then, using this guide, eliminate any products that don't fit your skin care or health goals. Be mindful that some products can be used for more than one purpose—for example, a lip balm can make a great cuticle conditioner. Some shampoos can be used as body wash, bar soaps can be used for shaving, and, to borrow an item from the kitchen, olive oil can be a good all-over moisturizer.

This book casts a wide net and covers many facets of skin care products, but each element is an important piece of the whole. You'll learn how to identify your skin's needs, how to address each need, and how to keep up with your skin's changes. You'll receive information on how to care for your skin, no matter your stage in life. Also included are 10 recipes for simple yet effective DIY products. Look forward to profound results!

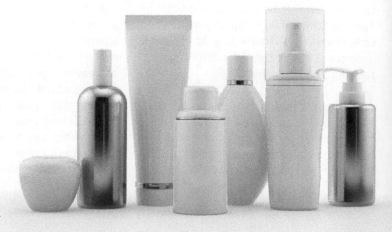

1

THE BUSINESS OF
Skin

1

THE BUSINESS OF
Skin

The average person has about 20 square feet (2 square meters) of skin covering their body. Skin shields us, surrounds us, and holds us together. It's a passageway to our bloodstream, and its appearance shapes our self-image. Here we'll discuss the basics about skin and how the beauty industry markets products to us.

YOUR LARGEST ORGAN

Weighing an average of 6 pounds (2.7 kilograms), your skin has two main layers: the epidermis (outer) and the dermis (inner). It also has the hypodermis. We'll take a closer look at these here.

Put simply, healthy skin is vital for our survival—both emotionally and physically. It is important to understand its role and relevance for our overall health, and to learn how to properly care for it.

- The hypodermis (right beneath the skin) is fat that pads and insulates.
- The dermis is the innermost layer of skin and contains nerve endings, sweat glands, hair follicles, and blood vessels that provide your skin with structure and support.
- The epidermis is the protective barrier. The cells in the epidermis are continually replaced by cells from the bottom layer. Your entire epidermis is replaced about every 27 days, although this process slows as we age.

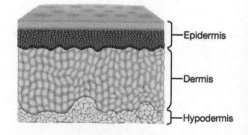

— Epidermis

— Dermis

— Hypodermis

THE ONE THING
YOU CAN'T LIVE WITHOUT

Our skin is something we often take for granted. It literally holds us together, protects us, and helps us maintain overall health. Caring for it is not only beneficial but is also vital, as we can't live without it.

Protective Barrier
Every day, our skin is bombarded by things it has to defend us from: chemicals in products we use, environmental toxins and pollutants, harmful bacteria, viruses, parasites, harmful pathogens, antigens, and UV radiation. And not only does our skin protect us from harmful elements that might otherwise gain access to our internal systems, it also must be healthy to preserve our internal fluids and organs.

Guarding Against Harm
The first place we feel pain and discomfort is the skin, which signals the brain that there is harm present—basic examples are stepping away from the heat of a fire before we can be burned, or moving away from the pressure of a sharp object before it cuts deeper. Therefore, our skin can tell us a lot about our health. Practitioners look at the skin for early warning signs as indicators for many diseases such as lupus, Lyme disease, and hepatitis C, which can first appear on our skin.

Comfort
Skin is your body's natural heating and air-conditioning system. It regulates temperature, helping avoid overheating or freezing by maintaining a consistent inner-body temperature regardless of the outside temperature.

Pleasure
Skin is key to so many aspects of our overall health. Touch brings us everything from a sense of well-being and comfort to feelings of happiness, joy, and titillation. There is nothing better than a hug from a loved one.

Who We Are
So much of how we feel about and how we perceive ourselves is wrapped up in our appearance. Beyond holding us together, our skin also influences our emotions. Those who treat individuals with skin ailments such as rosacea, acne, psoriasis, and eczema know the emotional effect our skin has on our well-being. It can make us depressed, unwilling to leave our homes and be around others, and can cause anxiety and stress and limit our social life. Yet when we see our skin conditions subside, we feel uplifted and can return to our regular lifestyles with a more positive attitude. Healthy skin helps us maintain our *overall* health.

THE MYTH OF SKIN TYPES

We have been taught to believe there are four basic skin types: normal, oily, dry, and combination. Truthfully, skin is dynamic! It changes constantly and can't be boxed in. You can wake up with dry skin and have oily skin by noon. You may have oily skin during your teen years and excessively dry skin as you age. But beyond skin type, it's more important to give your skin what it needs. While there are specific ingredients that target different skin types, there are also commonalities in certain ingredients that benefit all types of skin. Consider your facial moisturizer. All skin (even oily skin) needs to be moisturized with oils that are noncomedogenic, meaning they do not clog pores.

Often, skin types and tendencies such as acne, redness, and sensitivity are hereditary. Learning more about your parents' skin will be helpful as you maintain your own.

BIG BUSINESS

The personal care industry is one of the largest and fastest-growing industries. With a vast amount of money at stake, major companies and independent beauty businesses are constantly vying for a piece of the action. Along with this come big marketing budgets to entice you, the consumer, to spend your money. There are many conflicting messages, and much is at stake. Consumer education is key.

Label Smarts
Cutting through the jargon on the front of a product label (see page 5) and becoming

Common Skin Issues

Skin can be affected by a variety of issues, including blemishes, acne, eczema, psoriasis, redness or rosacea, sensitivity, hyperpigmentation, and seborrheic dermatitis. We'll review a few of them here, along with a few good-for-you ingredients that can work to clear these issues.

Blemishes, blackheads, and acne. Acne is evidence of inflamed or infected sebaceous glands and/or hair follicles.
<u>Try</u> activated bamboo or coconut hull charcoal and white willow bark.

Eczema/atopic eczema. This common skin condition causes patches of inflamed, rough, and cracked skin, and blisters that are sometimes itchy. Atopic eczema means the immune system has been affected.
<u>Try</u> bathing in colloidal oats and Dead Sea salt and using pure shea butter or avocado oil.

Psoriasis. This condition speeds up the life cycle of skin cells, causing them to build up very fast on the surface of your skin. These extra cells make scales and red patches.
<u>Try</u> bathing in colloidal oats and Dead Sea salt, using pure shea butter or avocado oil, and using salt scrubs.

Rosacea and redness. Rosacea causes facial blood vessels to enlarge, making the cheeks and nose flushed and red. Other issues can also cause redness, such as sensitivity, eczema, psoriasis, and acne.
<u>Try</u> neroli toner and facial mists, licorice root, and any oils with high essential fatty acid content.

General sensitivity. This issue is increasing across all age groups. Sensitivity can be caused by the products you use; exposure to sun, wind, and water; even polluted air. Reactions can include rashes and itching, redness, irritation, and burning.
<u>Try</u> olive, coconut, and avocado oils.

Hyperpigmentation In this case, patches of skin become a darker color than the rest of your skin. It often occurs when there is an excess of melanin—the substance that creates varying degrees of pigment.
<u>Try</u> raw potato, lemon juice, niacinamide, and turmeric.

Seborrheic dermatitis. This is generally seen on the scalp. It appears as scaly patches, dandruff, and redness. It can also be found in oily areas such as your face, sides of your nose, ears, eyebrows, chest, and eyelids.
<u>Try</u> coconut butter, olive leaf oil, and/or tea tree oil.

intimate with the ingredients is vital to understanding what you're putting on your skin. I recommend letting go of any associations you have about any particular brand being "natural" or "nontoxic." Many products have been "greenwashed" and sold in a certain way for so long we rarely stop to consider what's actually in them. "Greenwashing" is a term used to describe companies that make misleading or incorrect claims about the environmental benefits or health status of their product. Such claims can make a product seem more natural or environmentally friendly than it actually is. For example, "all natural," "eco-friendly," "Earth safe," and "hypoallergenic" suggest that the product is beneficial for consumers and the environment, but the terms are meaningless.

There are two important factors in determining whether a product is right for you. First, look at the ingredients, research them, and decide if they align with your health goals, and second—and most important—see how your skin reacts to them.

Let's take a look at a label for a common product. Note that ingredients are listed by their amounts, from largest to smallest.

Propylene glycol (vegetable derived)

Propylene glycol is a penetration enhancer, meaning it has the ability to cross the skin barrier and carry all the other chemicals in a product through the skin and into the bloodstream. It's a suspected immune system, reproductive, skin, and respiratory toxin. Used here, it gives the deodorant slickness to help it glide. Beyond that, there's no real efficacy. The "vegetable derived" simply serves to make us feel more comfortable about this ingredient, which may have been derived from vegetables but may also have been altered chemically for use here. Many other substances—wax and butter bases, for

example—are safer and offer the same efficacy.

Water

In general, water is a safe ingredient. However, once you formulate or add it to a product, you need a strong preservation system because, depending on its source, water can contain contaminants or heavy metals and is a breeding ground for bacteria, mold, and fungus.

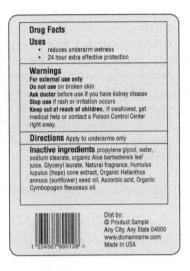

Drug Facts

Uses
- reduces underarm wetness
- 24 hour extra effective protection

Warnings
For external use only
Do not use on broken skin
Ask doctor before use if you have kidney disease
Stop use if rash or irritation occurs
Keep out of reach of children. If swallowed, get medical help or contact a Poison Control Center right away.

Directions Apply to underarms only

Inactive ingredients propylene glycol, water, sodium stearate, organic Aloe barbadensis leaf juice, Glyceryl laurate, Natural fragrance, Humulus lupulus (hops) cone extract, Organic Helianthus annuus (sunflower) seed oil, Ascorbic acid, Organic Cymbopogon flexuosus oil.

Dist by:
© Product Sample
Any City, Any State 04000
www.domainname.com
Made in USA

1 234567 890128 >

Sodium stearate

This is the sodium salt of stearic acid and can be variously sourced: coconut, palm oils, and lard, for example. It is often used to harden soap or deodorant.

Organic *Aloe barbadensis* leaf juice

This is a natural, wonderful ingredient for skin care purposes. However, many people have an allergy or sensitivity to it. Make sure you do a patch test.

Glyceryl laurate

Like propylene glycol, this is a penetration enhancer. It could easily have been omitted from this product and replaced with a natural ingredient, with less harm and more benefit. However, replacing it with a more beneficial alternative may increase the cost of the product.

Natural fragrance

Here "natural fragrance" is meaningless. In general, if a product is truly naturally scented, the label will specify the essential oils used. But because here it does not, this cannot be recommended as a safe ingredient. It's worth noting that there has been an industry push to make companies list all ingredients used in their scent blends, even though this is often considered proprietary information.

Humulus lupulus (hops) cone extract

Hops are commonly used as a calming, stress-relieving agent, but here we don't know what carrier the hops are extracted in and so cannot know if the carrier is beneficial or potentially harmful. Propylene glycol, for example, is a common carrier. Because the hops follow the fragrance in the listing, there's likely not a tangible amount of hop extract in the product.

Organic Helianthus annuus (sunflower) seed oil

A lovely ingredient, but due to its position on the ingredient list, it's unlikely there's any substantial amount present. This is likely a bit of "window dressing," in which an ingredient looks great on a label but there's not enough of it to have any real effect.

Ascorbic acid

Ascorbic acid is a vitamin C and a superstar ingredient in many skin care products. It is generally used in facial care products, as an antioxidant to prevent and reverse signs of aging.

Organic Cymbopogon flexuosus oil

This is a type of lemongrass essential oil. As the final ingredient, it's questionable how much is really in the product.

Overall, this is a really good example of the pitfalls of some "natural" products. Most of the work done to convince consumers is contained in the phrase "aluminum-free," a term most people are familiar with and an ingredient we're advised to avoid. After that, most consumers will assume everything else is safe. When you're considering what to buy, try to push past the advertising and get right to the label.

The 13 Unclean

There are 13 ingredients I believe we should avoid entirely—these aren't the only ones that should be avoided, but they are the top offenders. Try to avoid a product if you notice any of these ingredients near the beginning of the ingredients list. For more information on these, find their definitions in part 3 (page 17).

1. Parabens
2. Formaldehyde and formaldehyde donors
3. Phthalates
4. Diethanolamine and triethanolamine
5. Diazolidinyl urea and imidazolidinyl urea
6. Sodium lauryl sulfate/laureth sulfate; ammonium laureth sulphate
7. Propylene glycol
8. PVP/VA Copolymer
9. Nanoparticles
10. Synthetic fragrance (see Fragrance, page 56)
11. Triclosan
12. Toluene
13. Sunscreen chemicals

KNOWLEDGE IS POWER

Unless we educate ourselves, we are powerless against a billion-dollar industry that will do anything to sell us the latest miracle cure. Keep in mind, everyone has different needs and comfort zones in terms of what they use on their skin—some are perfectly comfortable using products that contain a lot of chemicals; others will not be. As long as you are an informed consumer, there is no right or wrong when it comes to choosing products. However, I do believe that in a virtually unregulated industry, consumers should take a "guilty until proven innocent" approach. I strongly advocate that all questionable ingredients be left out until ingredient manufacturers produce the information needed to let the consumer make choices they feel comfortable with. In order to make choices that fit within your personal criteria, you need to be educated. Otherwise, you risk allowing chemicals and toxins into your bloodstream, where they can affect your health without your consent or knowledge. I suggest you make your own criteria of what you will or won't use.

When we consider the impact beauty products can have on our appearance and health, we might think there would be stringent guidelines attached to bringing them to market. Unfortunately, there are not. Basic guidelines exist—such as guarding against outrageous health claims, a specific order of ingredients, and how the ingredients are listed—but these are relatively simple procedures to follow, making it easy for people to make and sell products. This can include individuals who have no experience with skin, ingredients, formulating, or sanitary and preservation practices. While it might seem easy to whip up simple products in the kitchen, there is a great deal involved in making a quality, truly beneficial product, so while I love supporting creativity and industriousness, I want everyone to be responsible about it. People have brought me homemade products for review and often they can have natural ingredients that can cause skin issues when used in the intended application. Additionally, not all ingredients work well together, and certainly not all "natural" ingredients are good for you. Tempering our enthusiasm with some structure would go a long way—and it can start with you being an actively informed consumer.

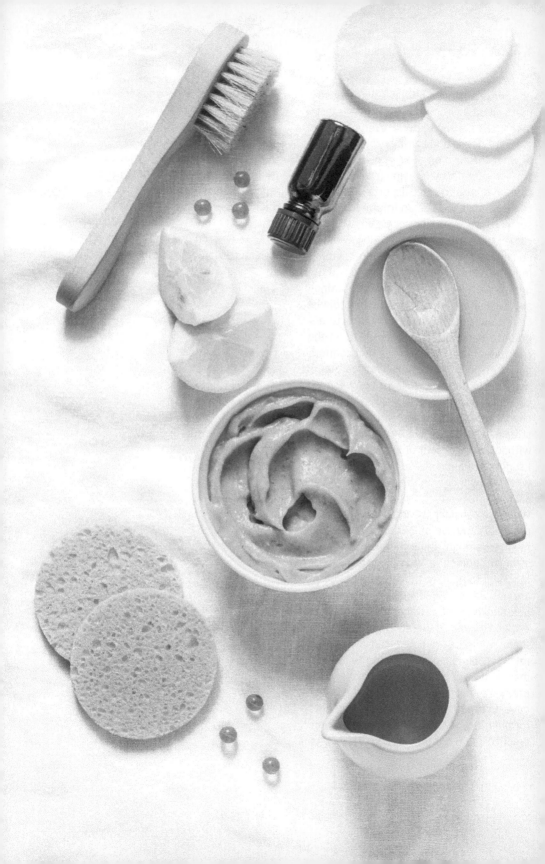

2 | CARING FOR YOUR
Skin

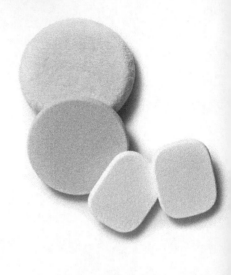

2 CARING FOR YOUR
Skin

Long ago, I realized that caring for skin involved more than just putting products on it. In 1998, while searching for a name for my company, I landed on "Sumbody." This name encompasses my beliefs about skin—that it's the sum of everything we do that keeps us healthy and glowing. From the food we eat to the thoughts we think, it all shows up on our skin. In this part, we'll discuss the full spectrum of caring for skin and highlight the different aspects.

TAKE CHARGE OF YOUR HEALTH

If any of my clients has been particularly indulgent, they tend to try and hide their face from me. I tell them everything shows up on the skin: the emotional residue of the fight with their significant other, excessive partying, lack of sleep, poor diet, and much more. I can see it all. They joke and say I'm psychic, but it's their skin that gives it away.

Eat Well, Look Good

We now know of the strong connection between diet and skin health. In fact, some of the very same things we use as skin care products are included in what I call a "beauty diet" composed of "beauty foods." In general, this involves eating as close to the earth as possible, or the way nature provided. This means not eating processed and condensed foods. For example, eating an apple rather than drinking apple juice. Apples contain fiber and other important nutrients and have a limited amount of sugar, whereas apple juice is high in sugar and doesn't contain all the other nutrients. Think fruits, vegetables, nuts, seeds, grains, legumes, etc.

An important aspect to the beauty diet is not only what you eat but also how you prepare and store your food. Use the right ingredients to do the right job—oils with high smoke points (such as avocado oil) are good for stir-fries and sautéing; olive oil is a perfect addition to salad dressings and cold dishes.

Simple changes you can make that are good for the environment and your overall health might be: using glass containers for food storage to reduce the amount of plastic your food is exposed to, drinking water out of glass or stainless steel, or buying or making produce storage bags from fabric.

The Probiotic Connection

When functioning properly, your immune system attacks anything in your body that it recognizes as a foreign contaminant, such as invading microbes, plant pollen, or chemicals. This process is called inflammation. Occasional inflammatory episodes targeting truly threatening invaders help fight off infection, protecting your health, including your skin. But sometimes inflammation can persist even when your body isn't under threat. At this point, inflammation can become the enemy rather than the protector. Many major diseases, including cancer, heart disease, diabetes, arthritis, depression, Alzheimer's disease, psoriasis, and chronic fatigue syndrome have been linked to chronic inflammation.

When I began my practice, I quickly noticed the connection between gut health, diet, and radiant skin. What you eat absolutely shows up on your skin. More and more doctors recognize this and are shifting their focus to what we put *in* our bodies rather

than *on* them. Our most valuable remedies, it turns out, may come from the farm, not the pharmacy!

The anti-inflammatory diet is growing in popularity among doctors and health care specialists for its benefit to your overall health. While it is more a lifestyle than a diet, these foods and guidelines not only reduce inflammation but also help maintain youthful, beautiful skin (see the sidebar on the next page). In addition to lowering inflammation, a more natural, less processed diet can have a positive influence on both your physical and emotional health. The foods and guidelines can be modified to fit almost any diet you adhere to. For example, the combination of growth hormones and inflammatory substances in many dairy products can, and often do, lead to acne. Other skin ailments, for example rosacea, are amplified by certain foods such as mint, alcohol, and spicy foods. It's all connected, and what you eat is reflected by your skin.

Vitamin J

I maintain that life is too short to completely abolish what you love. I live by what I call the 85/15 percent lifestyle. This means 85 percent of the time I eat a healthy diet, use healthy products, and think positive, healthy thoughts. The remaining 15 percent of the time, I have my vitamin J—junk. I indulge in an occasional cocktail, slice of pizza, scoop of ice cream, or highlight my hair. Having what you love from time to time increases the success rate of a major lifestyle change. Whatever your vitamin J is, or if there are deal breakers that you can't live without, relax. Indulge every now and then.

Exercise and Sleep

Sleep and exercise are also key factors in maintaining skin health. While you sleep, your skin cells are not—they are actively

Here are some simple shifts that can yield big results. In general, try to:

- Avoid processed foods; eat whole foods instead
- Drink lots of water
- Eat a variety of foods each meal and day
- Choose organic/fresh food whenever possible
- Eat a variety of whole grains
- Avoid canned foods
- Include a wide variety of beans
- Include winter squash, sweet potatoes, and avocados
- Eat the rainbow every day; plenty of fresh fruits and vegetables, not just the ones listed here

Inflammation Perpetrators

- Alcohol
- Artificial additives
- Bad fats (saturated, trans)
- Conventional meats and processed meats
- Dairy (unsweetened yogurt/kefir in moderation is fine)
- Excessive omega-6 fatty acids (in oils such as corn, safflower, grapeseed, peanut)
- Fast foods
- Fried foods
- Gluten and casein
- MSG
- Processed foods
- Refined carbohydrates
- Soda
- Sugar substitutes
- White sugar

Inflammation Fighters.

- Alliums: chives, garlic, leeks, onions, scallions, shallots
- Avocado
- Beans and legumes (best if soaked): black, chickpeas, lentils, navy, pinto, split peas, white
- Bee pollen
- Bone broth (for those who eat meat)
- Burdock root
- Cayenne powder
- Chocolate
- Cinnamon
- Cruciferous vegetables: bok choy, broccoli, Brussels sprouts, cabbage, cauliflower, collard greens, kale, radish, rutabaga, turnips, watercress
- Dark leafy greens
- Fruits: apples, blackberries, blueberries, cherries, citrus fruits, pineapple, raspberries, strawberries
- Ginger
- Green tea
- Oils: avocado, coconut, extra-virgin olive, walnut
- Omega-3s
- Seeds: chia, flax, pumpkin, sesame, sunflower
- Sprouted nuts and seeds: almond, cashew, hazelnut, macadamia, pecan, pistachio, walnut
- Sweet potatoes
- Turmeric
- Whole grains: amaranth, brown rice, buckwheat, oats
- Wild-caught fish high in omega-3: herring, mackerel, salmon, tuna (note: mercury and radiation issues are now a factor in how much fish to consume)
- Winter and summer squashes

Perfect Probiotics

Probiotics (good bacteria) are instrumental in maintaining good intestinal health. Plus, they help your colon get rid of toxic chemicals and pathogens.

- Kefir and coconut kefir
- Kimchi
- Kombucha
- Miso
- Pickles in their own brine
- Sauerkraut
- Tempeh

Prebiotics

Prebiotics nourish and feed the good bacteria in your colon. Both pre- and probiotics are imperative for a healthy gut.

- Alliums, raw: chives, garlic, leeks, scallions
- Apples
- Apple cider vinegar
- Avocado
- Bananas
- Chocolate (dark)
- Flaxseed
- Jerusalem artichokes
- Jicama
- Onions, raw and cooked
- Peas
- Wheat berries
- Wheat bran, raw
- Wheat germ

This list is just a starting place. Do what's healthy for you—omit anything you already know you are allergic to, and, if you have a medical condition that may prohibit any of these foods, check with your doctor before altering your diet.

regenerating. Cortisol (the stress hormone) surges during the day, and lack of good sleep can raise cortisol levels even further. Elevated cortisol levels cause inflammation, which, as we have learned, harms your skin. Think of it this way: All day long, your skin is protecting itself against constant attacks. At night, it finally has time to engage in intense repair, which is why it's so important to get good sleep. Human Growth Hormone (HGH), responsible for cell regeneration, also kicks in overnight. So does melatonin, which helps mend damage incurred during the day, increasing skin's ability to repair itself. Regular exercise contributes to skin health by improving circulation, enabling essential nutrients and oxygen to reach and nourish skin cells.

WHY DIY?

Making skin care products for your own use can be both fun and economical. With proper guidance and understanding, you can make effective products, know where your ingredients come from, use less packaging, and go preservative free. If you aren't convinced, here are two anecdotes.

A client was being cast on a TV show and had a sudden breakout. Since this client used my products, I was stumped as to what could be causing the problem. It turned out she had tried a popular DIY peeling face mask she found online—it was literally made of charcoal and white glue.

In another instance, a woman stopped in the shop to share some makeup she'd made from a recipe she found online. The color was lovely, and the ingredients were all natural, but overall the product was not good for skin—the combination of cinnamon, cornstarch, and cocoa powder may make for a delicious baked good, but cinnamon increases skin's photosensitivity.

I'm a big advocate for DIY, and there are 10 recipes for skin care products in part 4 (page 127), but be aware that information online is not always the best information. Here are some wonderful benefits of making products for your personal use.

Mind your budget. It's no secret that some skin care products come with big price tags. However, there are some products you can make that are just as effective as brand-name items, at a fraction of the cost. This is especially good for products you use frequently, like toners or masks. To further mitigate costs, consider asking a friend to co-op with you. You can buy ingredients in bulk to save money, but they won't go bad before you can use them. Beauty parties and DIY parties are fun ideas for making sure all the ingredients you purchase get used.

Set your own standards. Purchasing your own ingredients gives you the freedom and flexibility to customize products with exactly the ingredients you want and the ability to support companies you choose. You can use your purchasing power to support small, local, and/or organic farms and companies whose production and products align with your beliefs.

Keep things fresh. Some of the major offenders in over-the-counter (OTC) commercial products are the preservatives added to increase shelf life. By making small-batch products at home, you can use fresh ingredients and store your product on the shelf or in the refrigerator, eliminating the need for preservatives. You'll also be assured that you're using ingredients at the height of their potency.

Consider the environment. Use glass mason jars for salt scrubs, powdered face masks, bath salts, and body creams. Skip the middleman and eliminate all the cardboard boxes and hard plastic. Create less trash.

A SIMPLE SKIN CARE ROUTINE

A healthy skin care routine includes cleansing, toning, and moisturizing morning and night, using a serum if indicated/needed, and regular masks as needed. To establish a healthy routine, follow the steps below in the order they appear. If you use a mask, apply toner a second time after removing the mask.

Cleanse
It is imperative to cleanse the dirt, oil, and chemical buildup from your skin. Doing so allows other products to penetrate as well as waste to exit. Use your ring and middle finger to apply a small amount of cleanser, using small upward circular motions. Use light pressure (but not so light that you cannot feel it). Rinse with warm water (never hot water) by splashing water on your face until the cleanser is gone or use a soft clean washcloth.

Skin care products that contain chemicals ending in "-cone" (e.g., dimethicone, silicone) can actually form a plug in your pores; it's like putting caulk in your pores, which mixes with existing oil and dirt and makes that plug nearly impossible to pull out. If you use these products, you may need to cleanse more than once to loosen clogged and congested pores. Be patient: They are hard to remove. Double cleansing is recommended if you:
- Are exposed to air pollution daily
- Travel by plane or commute by car
- Smoke

- Horseback ride, garden, bike, or do anything that kicks up a lot of dirt/small particles
- Have excessively oily skin

Tone

Most people skip this step in their daily routine, but I suggest you don't. Toner rids your pores of the last traces of dirt and oil that the cleanser may have missed and prepares them for your moisturizer, which will be able to penetrate more deeply. Additionally, if your toner has effective "actives" (ingredients added for desired results, e.g., anti-acne or age defying), clean pores will allow these ingredients to penetrate even deeper. Toner should also balance your pH, which is a very important part of maintaining healthy skin.

To apply toner, use a cotton ball or soft cotton pad. Start at your neckline and move upward.

You only need to apply toner once unless you see dirt or cleanser on your pad or cotton ball. Reapply until the pad comes out clean.

Mask

Masks are another often overlooked step. I cannot stress enough how important they are; they truly are one of the workhorses of a good skin care system. Masks do everything from deep pore cleansing to helping get rid of dead skin cells to supplying vital nutrients and vitamins.

You may have been taught to let masks harden on your face and sit for a few minutes before removing them. It's time for a new tactic. "Hydrolizing" masks with passive steam allow the active ingredients in the mask to travel through your pores so the ingredients can actually have an effect. I prefer a powdered mask that is activated with water because every time you use it, it's at its peak potency and freshness. To apply a mask, use your fingers or a fan brush. Ideally, after application, take a shower as the steam level is perfect. Shower as normal and rinse off the mask at the end. If you prefer to take a bath, soak a hand towel in warm (not hot) water, wring it out, and place the towel over your face. For safety, leave your mouth and nose exposed. After the allotted time, remove the mask with the same towel, and do a quick water rinse.

Serum

Serums are problem solvers. If you have a specific skin issue (acne, excessive dryness, wrinkles, sagging, etc.) that you want to resolve, a targeted serum is a perfect choice. Not everyone needs serums; skip this step if it does not apply to you.

Before applying moisturizer, use your ring and middle finger to massage a small amount of serum onto your skin, making small upward circular motions.

If you have two separate issues you would like to address (e.g., wrinkles and dehydration), I suggest you work first on one and then focus on the other. Too many combined actives and products at once are not always beneficial.

Moisturize

All skin needs moisture. If you have oily skin, avoiding moisturizer will only cause your skin to overproduce oil to compensate. If you have dry skin, you can surely feel how you need moisturizer. However, not all moisturizers are meant for all types of skin. It is important to use the right one for your skin type.

Use your ring and middle finger to massage a small amount of moisturizer onto your skin, making small upward circular motions.

If your skin still feels dry after applying moisturizer, try doubling up to what I call "seal the deal." Use an oil-based face moisturizer and then layer a face cream

on top. This technique also works for dry skin on your body.

GO FORWARD IN GOOD HEALTH

Caring for your skin, learning about skin care ingredients, making your own products, and trying to figure out what you want to put on your skin can be daunting. My best advice is to do what feels right for you. If you prefer certain brands or certain ingredients, the definitions in part 3 will help you identify exactly what is in those products. If you're feeling adventurous and want to try DIY, you'll find 10 recipes in part 4 (page 127).

The beauty industry is changing because consumers are demanding it. Let your dollars send a powerful message—the more demands you make, the more changes we will see. People tell me they feel powerless to effect any change, but as an industry insider I can tell you that you are not powerless. It's because of you, the consumer, that there are now cleaner and healthier options available.

My hope is that you will use this guide to broaden your knowledge about the products you purchase and use on your skin. Knowledge is power!

3

INGREDIENT & TERM

Definitions

3 INGREDIENT &
Term Definitions

Having an understanding of the origins, uses, and benefits of products you use on your skin can help you determine if a particular ingredient falls in line with your goals and comfort level. There is a great deal of controversy about many ingredients; you can find some sources that say they are safe and others that say they are not. In the following definitions I try to refrain from giving my opinion. Instead, I simply provide you with the necessary information to make your own choices.

Note:
Terms in bold font within the definitions are cross-references to main entries.

1,2 hexanediol: Related to **propylene glycol**, this chemical is used as a preservative, thickening agent, filler, **humectant**, and conditioner. It carries the ingredients in a product through the skin barrier into the bloodstream. While there is no skin benefit, its low toxic rating means natural skin care companies use it as a preservative.

Acacia catechu gum: Also called cutch tree, this has historically been used in Ayurvedic medicine for skin ailments. It is also used as an astringent and for its consistency, viscosity, and texture.

Acacia concinna **bark extract:** **Saponins** in the bark of this Asian tree, also known as shikakai, make a very light lather when agitated or shaken with water. Rich in **antioxidants** and **vitamins A, D, C,** and **E,** the extract is used in skin cleansers and antiaging face creams.

Acacia concinna **fruit extract:** The dried acacia leaves and fruit are used in conditioners, facial cleansers, and shampoos.

Acacia decurrens **bark extract:** The rich tannin content in the bark of this Australian shrub, also known as green wattle, is added to cleansers, toners, and facial moisturizers. Gum is also made from the bark and used for viscosity and thickening.

Acacia decurrens **flower extract:** The extract from the acacia flowers, which contain a nutrient-dense pollen, is used in face creams targeting the effects of aging. The flowers are also made into a beautiful yellow dye that is useful as a natural colorant.

Acacia essential oil (*Acacia dealbata*): Also known as cassia, this oil has a mildly sweet, warm, calming scent and is widely used in body products and perfume. The essential oil comes from the extract of both the flowers and the leaves. It is suitable for all skin types and said to brighten dull skin.

Acacia farnesiana **flower extract** (*Vachellia farnesiana*): This extract is widely used in cosmetics to impart scent, but little research has been conducted about it.

Acacia farnesiana **gum** (*Vachellia farnesiana*): Also known as sweet acacia, this gum is used in cosmetics to control viscosity, for thickness, and as a binder.

Acacia farnesiana **root extract** (*Vachellia farnesiana*): The **antioxidants** in this root make the extract useful for the treatment of acne and aging skin.

Acacia flower extract (*Acacia dealbata*): This extract is used for skin conditioning and to calm and soothe sensitive, red, irritated skin.

Acacia flower wax (*Acacia dealbata*): Made from the flower solvent extraction, this wax is used as an emollient, thickening agent, and **emulsifier**.

Acacia leaf extract (*Acacia dealbata*): This extract is used for its restorative and protective properties, generally in antiaging products to soften and soothe skin and protect collagen.

Acacia seed extract (*Acacia dealbata*): Research has shown positive effects of this seed extract on the signs of aging. It helps repair and mend collagen, visibly reduce wrinkles, generate new skin cells, and protect skin from environmental damage. Effective when used alone, it is even more effective when used in conjunction with other active ingredients like **antioxidants** and **essential fatty acids**.

Acacia senegal gum extract (*Senegalia senegal*): Also known as gum arabic, this fiber-rich gum made from the sap is used to create viscosity and as a thickening agent in creams, lotions, and serums.

Acai berries (*Euterpe oleracea*): Grown by a tropical palm tree native to South and Central America, acai berries are very high in **antioxidants** and amino acids. Acai is frequently used in face creams, serums, and masks to combat a variety of skin concerns ranging from acne to aging. The berries can be used fresh; as an extract in either alcohol, glycerin, or solvent; or powdered.

Acai berry oil (*Euterpe oleracea*): Made from whole berries through a cold process, this very pure oil retains all the nutrients and vitamins of the whole berry. It has anti-inflammatory and antibacterial qualities and is rich in **essential fatty acids**. Light, nongreasy, and easily absorbed, it is used in face oils, creams, and serums targeting aging, acne, and dehydration.

Acai seed oil (*Euterpe oleracea*): The seeds of the acai fruit contain a rich and diverse selection of **essential fatty acids** and **antioxidants**. Oil from the seeds is powerfully anti-inflammatory and helps protect skin against environmental damage.

Activated coconut hull charcoal: This is one of the cleanest charcoals available. Millions of tiny pores help it adhere to and draw out toxins, oils, and buildup from skin pores. Its extraordinary cleaning ability enables proper skin functioning and leaves skin smooth and supple.

Agar agar: Derived from seaweed, agar agar takes on a gelatinous consistency when combined with water. It is a popular ingredient in DIY peeling masks and is used as a thickening agent in facial moisturizers, liquid soaps, and powders.

Agave (*Agave americana*): When used as a moisturizer, agave can protect skin from environmental damage, alleviate sunburn pain, and stimulate collagen production.

Agave leaf stem cell extract (*Agave americana*): Stem cell use is becoming very popular in skin care products. This extract can protect skin against environmental stress and sun damage. It is also a powerful ingredient in antiaging products.

Ajowan essential oil (*Trachyspermum ammi*): Also known as bishop's weed, this oil is extracted from the seeds of the ajwain plant, native to India. It has antibacterial, antiviral, antifungal, and antiseptic properties and is often used to treat skin infections and acne.

Alaea Hawaiian sea salt: This clean, pure sea salt is enriched with purified red volcanic alaea clay. The salt enhances the clay's mineral profile and its ability to clear clogged pores. It is used in detoxifying baths, foot soaks, exfoliating scrubs, and purifying products.

Alfalfa (*Medicago sativa*): Considered an herb but actually in the legume family, alfalfa is rich in vitamins (especially K), **saponins**, **flavonoids**, and amino acids. It is used in skin care to help retain moisture, give a nutrient boost, and treat acne and excessively dehydrated skin.

Allantoin: Found naturally in plants such as chamomile, comfrey, and sugar beet, allantoin is generally used in a synthetic form for cosmetic use. It is regarded as nonirritating and a highly effective moisturizing agent. It is often added to antiaging creams and used to treat dehydrated skin, psoriasis, and eczema.

Almond meal (*Oleum amygdalae*): Almond meal provides the same benefits as **almond oil** but in a less concentrated form. It is a gentle exfoliator often used in powdered masks, exfoliating powders, and body soap.

Almond oil (*Oleum amygdalae*): This common and cost-effective oil has high levels of **essential fatty acids** and **vitamin E**. It is often included in body lotions and face creams to help skin retain moisture and prevent fine lines and other signs of aging.

Aloe vera (*Aloe barbadensis*): This tropical evergreen, perennial succulent plant is a traditional remedy for many ailments and issues including sunburn, dry skin, and inflammation. Aloe contains enzymes that help exfoliate skin by encouraging cell renewal to combat aging. It is added to many products such as face creams, body lotions, toners, and after-sun gels.

Aloe vera butter (*Aloe barbadensis*): This butter is the extraction of **aloe vera** into fractionated coconut. It retains all the attributes of aloe vera but in a less concentrated form and is commonly used to form a creamy, smooth texture in body creams and lotions.

Aloe vera oil (*Aloe barbadensis*): This oil is similar to **aloe vera butter** but is extracted into a carrier oil that is liquid at room temperature, making it accessible for face care formulations.

Alpha hydroxy acids (AHAs): A group of synthetic and naturally derived active ingredients, AHAs include **glycolic, lactic, mandelic, tartaric, citric,** and **malic acids.** AHAs are popular for their ability to exfoliate dead skin cells; smooth wrinkles and fine lines; improve elasticity, texture, and tone; clean pores; and resurface skin. They are also said to be effective at acne scar removal and skin lightening. The level of exfoliation depends on the type and amount of AHAs used. In some professional applications where an alpha hydroxy peel is used, some people report redness, sensitivity, and irritation. Natural AHA products and chemical peels differ in intensity and efficacy. AHAs cause photosensitivity.

Alpha-lipoic acid: This effective **antioxidant** enzyme is often mixed with other antioxidants in products targeting aging and congested pores. Most forms are a 50:50 mix of synthetic and natural components. Often used in serums, it efficiently penetrates skin and effectively reduces wrinkles and fine lines, restores glow, and prevents signs of aging.

Aluminum chlorohydrate/chloride: Created by reacting aluminum with hydrochloric acid, this inorganic salt can alter skin pH balance and reduce sweat production, making it an effective ingredient in antiperspirants and deodorants. Many believe that topical application of aluminum salts can lead to breast cancer and Alzheimer's disease, though there is no conclusive scientific evidence for either claim.

Aluminum oxide/alumina: Primarily used as a thickening agent that also aids in anticaking and absorption, this compound is frequently mixed into mineral powder makeup. It doesn't penetrate skin and the FDA (Food and Drug Administration) considers it safe for cosmetic use.

Amaranth flour (*Amarantus*): This is used in face care products as a gentle **exfoliant** that also offers **antioxidants** and collagen-boosting ingredients.

Amaranth oil (*Amarantus*): One of the best natural sources of squalene (a hydrator found naturally in skin), amaranth oil mimics sebum to help skin retain moisture and is a highly effective **emollient** and **antioxidant.** Increasingly popular for use in antiaging face creams, it is also said to be anti-inflammatory and antibacterial.

Amargo wood extract (*Quassia amara*): Derived from a small South American evergreen tree, this extract contains antiviral, anti-inflammatory, antifungal, insecticidal, and **antioxidant** properties. It is used to treat acne, as a conditioning agent in cosmetics, and traditionally to eradicate lice.

Amazonian lily extract (*Victoria amazonica*): Derived from an Amazonian water lily, this extract's high tannin content makes it an excellent astringent, working to minimize pores. Its rich composition of starch, glucose, and oils moisturizes, detoxifies, and nourishes skin for a smooth and supple appearance.

Amber extract: Amber is a naturally found resin, and the extract is lauded for its youth-preserving and cell-rejuvenating properties. The antiaging benefits are attributed to the high concentration of a powerful **antioxidant**. The ingredient is relatively new in high-end face care products, although amber has long been used as a scent.

American ginseng (*Panax quinquefolius*): Commonly used in Chinese medicine, ginseng's **phytonutrient**-rich roots and leaves are increasingly used in products for their antiaging properties. It is also used for skin brightening.

Ammonium lauryl sulfate (ALS): Derived from coconut or synthesized in a lab, this substance is a foaming agent popular for shampoos, body washes, and facial cleansers. ALS doesn't penetrate skin and hair as easily as smaller-molecule **surfactants** such as sodium laureth sulfate. Some believe this makes it a safer alternative. Considered an irritant at concentrations of 2% and above, it's regarded as safe for use in cosmetics but only in products designed for brief use followed by thorough rinsing.

Amyris essential oil (*Amyris balsamifera*): All parts of this bushy tree native to Haiti are used medicinally, topically, and aromatherapeutically. The oil, extracted from the wood, has antiseptic, anti-inflammatory, and sedative properties, and promotes skin regeneration while calming and reducing redness.

Amyris hydrosol (*Amyris balsamifera*): This hydrosol has all the benefits of the essential oil but in a less concentrated form so it can be used undiluted. It is added to cleansers and toners to keep pores clean, remove dead skin cells, and reduce inflammation.

Andiroba extract (*Carapa guianensis*): This extract can be powder or liquid. The liquid is generally extracted into an alcohol solvent. It has antiviral, antibacterial, and anti-inflammatory properties and is generally used in salves for muscle and joint aches and pains, and for treating wounds. It is also added to soap, face masks, and face and body scrubs as an **exfoliant**.

Andiroba oil (*Carapa guianensis*): Derived from the seeds of an Amazonian rainforest tree, this oil contains **essential fatty acids**, vitamins, and minerals. It is used in products targeting acne as well as in soap and natural insect repellents.

Anise essential oil (*Pimpinella anisum*): Anise essential oil is generally added to lotions, creams, bath salts, and soaps for its aroma, but its antiseptic property makes it useful in deodorants and hand sanitizers.

Anise seed extract (*Pimpinella anisum*): Native to the Mediterranean and Asia, anise is a flowering plant in the carrot family. Apart from its culinary uses, it is antimicrobial and an **antioxidant**. It is used topically to treat acne and to slow signs of aging.

Angelica essential oil (*Angelica archangelica*): Extracted from the angelica root, the oil is used in massage oils and bath salts to promote detoxification, treat psoriasis, and reduce inflammation. It can cause photosensitivity, so it should not be used in a strong concentration in skin care products.

Angelica hydrosol (*Angelica archangelica*): This hydrosol has all the benefits of the essential oil but in a less powerful form so it will not cause photosensitivity. It is used in baths to alleviate psoriasis, inflammation, and menstrual cramps.

Angelica leaf extract (*Angelica archangelica*): This extract is rich in tannins and is often used in combination with the root extract in cleansers and toners targeting the effects of aging.

Angelica root extract (*Angelica archangelica*): Traditionally used for treating ailments such as colds and the flu, and to boost the immune system and promote digestion, angelica is used topically to protect skin against pathogens and to help keep pores clean and clear.

Angelica seed (*Angelica archangelica*): Filled with **essential fatty acids** and antiseptic properties, these powdered seeds are used in face masks and **exfoliants**, or as an oil in face creams and face oils targeting dehydration.

Anthocyanins: Anthocyanins are natural plant pigments that produce red, blue, and purple colors. Their anti-inflammatory and **antioxidant** properties make them effective at wound healing, healthy cell regeneration, and increased production of collagen. They also protect skin against environmental damage and aging and are used in products targeting aging and acne.

Antioxidants: These substances are some of the mainstay ingredients in skin care products. Extensive studies have proven their ability to protect skin cells from sun damage, pollutants, and other factors that damage and kill cells. Antioxidants are not limited to but include **vitamins E and C**, **green tea**, **resveratrol**, and coenzyme Q10. They are effective for skin when used both topically and internally.

Apple (*Malus pumila*): This fruit is rich in **antioxidants**, vitamins, and the exfoliant **malic acid**. Apples are a prebiotic that feeds probiotics. Maintaining a flourishing population of beneficial flora on the skin surface is important for healthy skin.

Apple cider vinegar (ACV): The main ingredient of apple cider vinegar is acetic acid, although it also contains other acids (**lactic**, **citric**, and **malic**), vitamins, mineral salts, and amino acids. The acids "digest" dead skin cells, causing a mild cell turnover to reveal more vibrant, youthful, and healthy skin. With a pH similar to skin, ACV helps restore and balance the natural pH and acid of the skin's surface. It should always be diluted in purified water before applying.

Apple stem cell extract (*Malus pumila*): This extract contains powerful **antioxidants** that protect against signs of aging. While more research is being done on stem cells and skin care, apple stem cell extract is already being used more widely.

Apricot oil (*Prunus armeniaca*): Pressed from apricot seed, this oil is light and easily absorbed with no greasy residue. Rich in **antioxidants** and **vitamins A and E**, and containing **gamma linoleic acid**, it firms, moisturizes, hydrates, tones, soothes, and slows signs of aging. It is suitable for sensitive skin. It is used in products that treat acne as it has an anti-inflammatory effect, and it can reduce and clear breakouts. It is commonly found in body scrubs, lotions, oils, face creams, and face oils.

Apricot seed/kernel (*Prunus armeniaca*): This hard seed is finely milled into powder and added to facial scrubs as a facial **exfoliant**. Although the powder feels very fine, the kernel does not dissolve in water and retains jagged edges that can cause microdermabrasions.

Argan oil (*Argania spinosa L.*): Produced by cold-pressing the seeds of the argan tree native to Morocco, this oil is full of **vitamin E** and other **antioxidants**. Rich in **essential fatty acids**, it softens skin, increases elasticity, and reduces the appearance of wrinkles. It helps balance skin's natural oil production, is non-comedogenic, and is used to prevent breakouts. Argan oil has become a highly popular ingredient in skin and hair care products.

Arnica flower (*Arnica montana*): This perennial plant has long been used in homeopathic preparations and topically in ointments for bruises, sprains, arthritis, pain, and inflammation. It works gently to reduce redness and calm irritated skin, properties that make it effective for both antiaging and acne skin care. It is also used in bath salts and soaks.

Arrowroot: Derived from the rhizomes of different tropical plants, this very fine, soft, and silky powder can effectively replace cornstarch and is found in many products such as body powders, makeup, face masks, and creams for its ability to draw, absorb, and thicken.

Asafoetida essential oil (*Ferula foetida*): Made from both the root and stem of perennial herbs, this essential oil has antifungal, antiviral, and antibacterial properties effective for treating acne.

Asafoetida powder (*Ferula foetida*): Made from the rhizome of several species of perennial herbs, asafoetida has anti-inflammatory, antiviral, antibacterial, **antioxidant**, and sedative properties and is used in face masks and **exfoliants** that

are used for acne prevention, skin lightening, and treating the effects of aging. The powder is increasingly popular in natural skin care, as being able to make products without water eliminates the need for preservatives.

Ascorbyl palmitate: This synthetic, nonacidic form of **vitamin C** is often found in facial serums. Sometimes marketed as "vitamin C ester," it's formed from ascorbic acid and palmitic acid (a fatty acid from plants or animals). Because it is fat-soluble, it penetrates skin more easily than other forms of vitamin C. It's particularly effective at reducing environmental skin damage when applied topically. It can, however, increase photosensitivity.

Ashwagandha (*Withania somnifera*): The powdered root of this perennial shrub is commonly used in Ayurvedic medicine. There is little research on ashwagandha's topical benefits. Full of **flavonoids** that may rejuvenate skin cells, ashwagandha can be found in skin care products such as toners, serums, moisturizers, and eye creams.

Astragalus leaves (*Astragalus membranaceus*): Astragalus leaves are less commonly used internally than the root, although topically the leaves are used to increase the levels of **hyaluronic acid**, protect skin from cellular damage, maintain healthy collagen, and prevent aging.

Astragalus root (*Astragalus membranaceus*): This has been used for centuries in Chinese medicine to maintain a healthy immune system. Topically, its **antioxidant** benefits help strengthen skin cells, protect against damage, and ward off bacteria and viruses.

Astringent: An astringent is something that causes the contraction of body tissue, typically the skin. Astringents are generally found in toners marketed to reduce pore size and to cleanse and refresh skin. Pores, however, are not muscles and cannot expand and contract. Once they have been overstretched, they do not shrink back.

Avocado (*Persea americana*): High in **essential fatty acids**, vitamins, and minerals, avocados are gentle enough for all skin types. They protect, mend, and repair skin as well as moisturize and hydrate. Fresh avocados are used as face masks, and powdered avocado is added to increasing numbers of skin care products. Since there is no water in powdered avocado, it can be mixed with other ingredients such as clays and milks to make a powdered face mask without the need for preservatives.

Avocado butter (*Persea americana*): This is not a true plant butter but a combination of avocado oil and a hydrogenated vegetable oil. It has a rich, creamy texture and offers a different profile than the oil for products such as body creams, body lotions, bar lotions, soaps, and hand and foot balms.

Avocado oil (*Persea americana*): Much more concentrated than the fruit, avocado oil is extracted from the pulp and is rich in **essential fatty acids**, vitamins, **antioxidants**, and nutrients, making it beneficial for extremely dry and aging skin. It is noncomedogenic and leaves no greasy residue. Beneficial for irritated or sensitive skin, it soothes symptoms of psoriasis and eczema. The oil also increases collagen production and decreases inflammation.

Babassu seed oil (*Orbignya oleifera*): The edible oil is derived from the fatty seeds of the Amazonian babassu palm. Rich in **antioxidants** and **essential fatty acids**, it also has antifungal, antiviral, and anti-inflammatory properties. Although fairly rich and viscous, it quickly absorbs into skin. It is often used in products that target acne, severe dehydration, and premature aging, as well as in cuticle conditioners, bath oils, soaps, and massage oils.

Babchi leaf extract (*Psoralea corylifolia*): The extract of the Babchi leaf is rich in **antioxidants**, is an anti-inflammatory, and helps relieve stress. It is used in products such as face creams, bath soaks, and salves to promote relaxation, ease pain, treat psoriasis, and slow signs of aging.

Babchi seed oil (*Psoralea corylifolia*): These seeds come from an annual plant that grows in India, Africa, and China. Research has indicated efficacy in treating psoriasis, environmental damage, and signs of aging. It is used in face creams to reduce the effects of aging, in bath soaks and creams for psoriasis, and in massage oils and body lotions.

Bacillus coagulans: Part of the probiotic family, this bacteria is currently a hot ingredient in skin care products for acne, rosacea, eczema, and premature aging.

Bakuchiol: An extract derived from the seeds and leaves of **babchi**, bakuchiol is the new must-have ingredient in products for antiaging. Considered the new **retinol**, it is used for its ability to provide all the attributes of retinol but in a gentler formulation.

Balsam fir essential oil (*Abies balsamea*):
This astringent has antibacterial properties, so it is often used in rubs for congestion and steams for the relief of cold and flu symptoms. It is also used in hand sanitizers, soaps, hair care, and toners and for its aroma in scent blends.

Balsam of Peru essential oil (*Myroxylon balsamum*): Derived from a tree native to tropical South and North America forests, the **antioxidant**, anti-inflammatory, antibacterial, and antiseptic properties in this essential oil make it useful in deodorants and antiperspirants. It is an extremely concentrated essential oil used in very small amounts in massage oils for damaged and severely dry skin.

Bamboo charcoal (*Bambuseae*): The high surface-to-weight ratio of this charcoal makes it an excellent purifier that penetrates deeply into pores and draws out rancid oils, dirt, and impurities, detoxifying and allowing skin to breathe and function properly.

Bamboo leaf extract (*Bambuseae*): Bamboo leaf extract has **antioxidant** compounds that strengthen collagen structure, regenerate cells, visibly reduce wrinkles, and tone skin, making it beneficial in skin care products targeting mature skin.

Bamboo powder (*Bambuseae*): Very fine and rich in minerals and silica, bamboo powder is used in facial **exfoliants**, body powders, and makeup.

Bamboo vinegar (*Bambuseae*): Relatively new in skin care, this vinegar has antibacterial, antiviral, and antifungal properties that reduce redness, irritation, and itching, and eliminate dead skin cells and foot odor. It is used in facial toners and cleansers targeting acne, and also in foot soaks.

Banana (*Musa sapientum, Musa nana*):
Originally found in Malaysia, bananas are high in **vitamins B6** and **C**, manganese, potassium, and natural sugars that gently exfoliate and moisturize. They are effective at treating psoriasis and are most commonly used in powdered or extract form in skin care products, bath soaks, and face creams targeting dehydrated, irritated, aging, and psoriasis-prone skin.

Banana peel extract (*Musa sapientum, Musa nana*): The cosmetic industry started using banana peel extract for its amino acid, **antioxidant**, and sugar content. The extract is used in facial cleansers, **exfoliants**, and face creams. While rich in nutrients, it is gentle on skin and calms rashes, insect bites, and psoriasis.

Baobab (*Adansonia*): This tree grows in Australia, the Middle East, and parts of Africa. The fruit and seeds are used fresh or dried, or made into extract. It is said to have anti-inflammatory, antiviral, and antimicrobial properties as well as a high **vitamin C** content. When used topically, it visibly improves skin elasticity, helps prevent signs of aging, and acts as a natural moisture barrier.

Barberry (*Berberis vulgaris*): Traditionally, the fruit, bark, and berries of this European shrub have been used topically for their anti-inflammatory, antibacterial, antiviral, and antifungal properties. Barberry contains **berberine**, which not only kills bacteria and is anti-inflammatory but also is a mild sedative and immune-system booster. Barberry is used in skin care products to treat acne as well as in creams and salves for pain and fungal infections.

Bay essential oil (*Laurus nobilis*): This oil is antiseptic, antifungal, and anti-inflammatory and is used to treat acne and oily skin conditions. It is also added to perfumes and essential oil blends for scenting bath and body care products and soaps.

Bay hydrosol (*Laurus nobilis*): Bay hydrosol has all the properties of the essential oil but is less caustic. It is used in acne toners, acne cleansers, foot soaks, deodorants, and muscle sprays.

Bee pollen: Honeybees form tiny pellets of pollen held together by plant nectar and bee enzymes. The pollen is a power-packed nutrient-dense ingredient that aids in collagen production, visibly accelerates cell turnover, combats acne, and restores vibrancy to skin.

Beefsteak plant leaf extract (*Perilla ocymoides*): Extracted in various solvents, which make its purity range from below average to good, this leaf extract is filled with **antioxidants** and anti-inflammatories.

Beefsteak plant oil (*Perilla ocymoides*): The oil extracted from the beefsteak plant seed has antibacterial and anti-inflammatory properties as well as **essential fatty acids**. It helps gently remove dirt and oils from skin and is used in many products, from cleansers to face moisturizers. It can cause some sensitivity.

Beefsteak plant seed extract (*Perilla ocymoides*): Extracted in various solvents or powdered, the seeds from this plant native to Asia have antibacterial, antiviral, and antifungal properties.

Beet sugar: White table sugar comes from sugarcane or beets, the difference being how it is processed and refined. White sugar is processed with bone char to whiten the crystals, while beet sugar is not. Both are a natural form of **glycolic acid**, which gently exfoliates. Beet sugar also is a moisturizer that maintains intracellular hydration and helps prevent the damage and dehydration responsible for parched, sallow, and discolored skin.

Behenic acid: A fatty acid derived from plant oil extracts such as **moringa oil** and **pracaxi oil**. As a conditioning agent, it works to smooth hair follicles. It's also used as a thickening agent, surfactant, and opacifier. It's found in a wide range of products including hair care, deodorants, eyeliners, moisturizers, cleansers, and styling gels.

Behentrimonium chloride: Derived from **canola oil**, this substance has powerful conditioning properties, and its waxy texture makes it a popular ingredient in defrizzing hair products. It can also act as a preservative. The Environmental Working Group (EWG) rates it as 3/10, and it is Whole Foods Premium Body Care approved, but it is considered toxic in concentrations of 0.1% and higher. Conditioning agents are often highly toxic, and behentrimonium chloride is generally regarded as a safer option.

Bentonite clay: This highly absorbent clay is great for oily skin due to its ability to easily adhere to and draw out excess oil and toxins when mixed with water. Known for its toning, tightening, blemish-banishing, and pore-purging abilities, it is one of the most common and easily accessible clays.

Benzoin: A balsamic resin derived from a solvent extraction of the bark of several species of trees in the Styrax genus, benzoin is used in perfumes, incense, and essential oil blends. It is also used for wound healing, canker sores, and pain.

Benzoyl peroxide: This medicine kills the bacteria that cause acne. It also helps keep pores clear.

Berberine: An alkaloid found in plants and used internally in traditional Chinese medicine, berberine is an anti-inflammatory used in antiaging skin care products and in products targeting joint and muscle pain and inflammation.

Bergamot essential oil (*Citrus bergamia*): Bergamot is possibly a hybrid of lemon and bitter orange. The essential oil is antiseptic and bacterial and is added to deodorants and used to treat acne, athlete's foot, eczema, infections, fungal infections, inflammation, and psoriasis.

Bergamot hydrosol (*Citrus bergamia*): Bergamot hydrosol contains all the attributes of the essential oil in a less expensive form, which can be used undiluted or to replace water in products targeting acne, psoriasis, and eczema, and in facial toners, foot soaks, body sprays, and natural deodorants.

Bergamot juice (*Citrus bergamia*): Bergamot juice is rich in **antioxidants** and natural fruit sugars. It is used in facial cleansers to gently exfoliate and protect skin against environmental damage.

Bergamot leaf extract (*Citrus bergamia*): Bergamot leaves were traditionally applied directly to pimples to relieve breakouts. The leaf extract is now used in cleansers, toners, face creams, and serums to treat acne.

Beta hydroxy acid: Also known as salicylic acid, this comes from the bark of the white willow tree. Beta hydroxy acid is oil soluble, allowing it to deeply penetrate pores and rid them of congestion and buildup, unlike **alpha hydroxy acids**, which cannot penetrate the sebum (skin's natural oil) in pores. It also has anti-inflammatory and antibacterial properties and is therefore generally used in products designed to treat acne.

Beta-carotene: This yellowish-orange pigment is found in colorful fruits and vegetables, especially carrots. It is a provitamin that can be converted into active **vitamin A** and is a **carotenoid** and **antioxidant**. It can be used to fight free radical damage, increase collagen production, repair skin, and protect it from premature aging.

Betel leaf (*Piper betle*): These leaves come from a tropical evergreen vine and contain **beta-carotene**, **antioxidants**, tannins, and anti-inflammatory properties. Betel leaf helps protect skin against UV damage and maintains healthy collagen and skin structure.

Bilberry extract (*Vaccinium myrtillus* L.): Native to North America, Western Asia, and some parts of Europe, bilberry is filled with **anthocyanins** and **bioflavonoids** that protect against and reverse skin damage caused by free radicals and environmental toxins. It helps deliver oxygen-rich blood to the skin, which helps maintain elasticity and suppleness and aids in balancing the skin's natural oil production. It is often used in face creams, lotions, and makeup.

Bioflavonoid: Bioflavonoids are plant-derived compounds with powerful **antioxidant** properties.

Birch bark extract (*Betula alba*): Detoxifying, purifying, calming, healing, and mildly astringent, birch bark extract enables congestion in pores to be loosened and removed. Its anti-inflammatory properties soothe irritated skin and combat eczema and psoriasis.

Birch essential oil (*Betula alba*): Extracted from leaves and buds, birch essential oil is used to treat joint and muscle pain, as a mild astringent in skin care, and to treat psoriasis and eczema.

Birch hydrosol (*Betula alba*): Birch hydrosol has the same benefits as the essential oil but in a less caustic form, so it can be used undiluted. It is used in acne toners, in body creams to ease joint pain, compresses for sore muscles and pain, and in the bath to reduce joint and muscle pain.

Birch leaf extract (*Betula alba*): Birch buds and leaves are used for the extract, which is rich in **flavonoids, saponins**, and tannins. It is antifungal, antibacterial, antiviral, anti-inflammatory, and mildly astringent. It is used in products aimed at antiaging, brightening, and purifying.

Black cumin oil (*Nigella sativa*): Also known as black seed oil, black onion seed oil, or black caraway oil. The seeds are rich in **antioxidants**, minerals, and vitamins and are believed to have antibacterial, antiviral, anti-inflammatory, and antiseptic properties. In skin care the oil is most commonly used for acne, psoriasis, and dehydrated and aging skin. The National Psoriasis Foundation recommends using the oil both topically and orally to treat psoriasis.

Black currant bud floral wax (*Ribes nigrum*): This wax is used as an **emulsifier**, thickening agent, and **emollient** and to provide a smooth texture. It has astringent properties.

Black currant leaf extract (*Ribes nigrum*): Black currant leaves contain antibacterial, antiviral, anti-inflammatory, and antifungal properties. The extract is used to treat wounds, cuts, scrapes, insect bites, and joint pain. It is added to products such as salves and bath soaks for pain relief and wound healing.

Black currant seed oil (*Ribes nigrum*): Native to Europe and Asia, black currants contain a high concentration of **antioxidants, gamma-linolenic acid, essential fatty acids, vitamins A, B**, and **E**, and are a superstar source of **vitamin C**. The National Psoriasis Foundation recommends using the oil both orally and topically for psoriasis. It is beneficial for dry, itchy, and painful skin.

Black Hawaiian salt: This is not a true black salt but sea salt combined with activated charcoal made from the hulls of Hawaiian coconuts, which provide its color. With the addition of coconut charcoal, this salt is widely used for detoxifying baths, foot soaks, exfoliating scrubs, and purifying products.

Black musli (see *Curculigo orchioides*)

Black pepper essential oil (*Piper nigrum*): Black pepper comes from a vine native to India. The essential oil is rich in phytochemicals and has **antioxidant**, antibacterial, antifungal, and anti-inflammatory properties that are used in essential oil blends and perfumes. It protects against damage from UV rays and is a prebiotic, helping maintain a healthy microbiome.

Black pepper, ground (*Piper nigrum*): Ground black pepper has all the attributes of the essential oil but in a less caustic form. It is used as an **exfoliant** in facial scrubs, body scrubs, and bar soap.

Black raspberry seed oil (*Rubus occidentalis*): Extracted from black raspberry seeds in a cold-process method, this extremely pure oil contains high levels of **antioxidants** and **essential fatty acids**, has anti-inflammatory properties, and is used to protect skin against sun and environmental damage. It is a light, easily absorbed, nongreasy, noncomedogenic oil used in sunscreens and for dry, damaged, prematurely aging skin.

Black tea (*Camellia sinensis*): Brewed black tea can replace water in formulations to increase efficacy. Replacing water with other fluids such as hydrosols and teas is an effective way to impart active ingredients. Black tea is also used in soapmaking.

Black tea extract (*Camellia sinensis*): Filled with **antioxidants**, this extract is a staple in skin care formulations that target the prevention and reversal of aging.

Black or chebulic myrobalan (*Terminalia chebula Retz*): This whole plant is used to treat many ailments in Ayurvedic medicine. It has **antioxidant**, anti-inflammatory, antibacterial, and antiviral properties. Applied topically, it protects the skin's natural barrier, warding off toxins and germs. It is used to treat acne and dandruff, and added to salves and creams for foot care.

Black willow bark (*Salix nigra*): Black and white willow bark contain salicin and anti-inflammatory **flavonoids** beneficial for many skin ailments. The bark is a powerful ally against the appearance of aging skin. It is also used to decongest pores, smooth texture, prevent blemishes, and relieve pain; in acne products and antiaging products; and in muscle balms and pain-relieving bath soaks.

Blackberry (*Rubus allegheniensis*): Blackberries are filled with minerals and vitamins and are a particularly high source of **vitamin C**. When used in skin care they are concentrated, making the vitamin C levels profound. Blackberry regenerates skin cells and protects against environmental damage. It can be used either fresh or powdered and is becoming increasingly popular in skin care products.

Blackberry seed oil: This oil has all the benefits of the fruit with the addition of **essential fatty acids**. It is a noncomedogenic, easily absorbed, versatile oil that can be used in products ranging from face creams and oils to body lotions and serums.

Blue Cambrian montmorillonite: Rich in trace minerals, this highly absorbent clay is used for drawing out congestion in pores, to detoxify, and to combat acne and oily skin.

Blue lotus floral extract (*Nymphaea caerulea*): This extract is used for its ability to moisturize. It also helps balance the skin's natural oil production, so it is used to reduce and prevent acne breakouts, in antiaging skin products, and also as a calming, relaxing agent.

Blue lotus floral wax (*Nymphaea caerulea*): This floral wax has anti-inflammatory and **antioxidant** properties. It is an **emulsifier**, imparts viscosity, and creates an even, creamy texture. Its hydrating and oil-balancing benefits make it widely used in products targeting aging and acne.

Blue-green algae (*Cyanobacteria*): This microscopic organism lives in lakes, ponds, and streams. Packed with amino and fatty acids, the building blocks of healthy collagen and skin, it helps retard signs of aging and visibly lifts and tones skin, making it look rejuvenated.

Blueberry seed oil (*Vaccinium ssp*): Blueberries are considered a superfood, but their seed oil is also a powerhouse for skin. Rich in **antioxidants**, **essential fatty acids**, vitamins, and **phytonutrients**, this easily absorbed, nongreasy, and noncomedogenic oil is suitable for all skin types. It rejuvenates skin, restoring luster.

Bog bilberry (*Vaccinium myrtillus* L.): This member of the bilberry family contains one of the richest sources of **anthocyanins**, giving it its color and a significant **antioxidant** content. It is also anti-inflammatory. It protects collagen, promotes new cell growth, prevents the appearance of wrinkles and fine lines, and helps improve hydration levels.

Bolivian rose salt: This rare salt is hand-mined from ancient deposits in the Bolivian Andes Mountains. The mountains protected the salt from contaminants, conserving the abundant trace minerals that give it its unique color and ingredient profile. It nourishes, detoxifies, smoothes, remineralizes, and tones skin.

Borage oil (*Borago officinalis*): This oil is pressed from the seeds of the borage plant, which contain **essential fatty acids** that play a key role in healthy skin structure and function. It is noncomedogenic and creates a gentle skin barrier that conditions excessively dry skin. It is a delicate oil with a shelf life of about six months.

Boron nitride: A naturally occurring mineral powder that can also be synthesized, boron nitride is added to makeup and sunscreens to help other ingredients spread over skin. It also promotes adhesion and absorbs oil. Its crystalline structure refracts light from skin, giving a smooth, even-toned appearance. It's widely regarded as nontoxic and safe for cosmetic use.

Boysenberries (*Rubus ursinus x Rubus idaeus*): Rich in **antioxidants**, especially **vitamin C** and natural fruit sugars, boysenberries can be used fresh or powdered and are used in face masks, cleansers, and face creams that target the effects of aging before wrinkles appear. They also gently remove dead skin cells and help eliminate pore congestion.

Boysenberry seed oil: The cold-pressed oil from boysenberry seeds are high in **antioxidants** and **vitamins A, C, and E**. It protects skin from environmental damage and rejuvenates skin cells and collagen. The cold-pressed oil is not to be confused with the fragrance oil, which should be listed differently on the label as it is not derived from the berry.

Brazil nut oil (*Bertholletia excelsa*): This oil from the nuts of a tree native to South America is rich in selenium, **vitamin E**, **essential fatty acids**, and has anti-inflammatory and antiaging properties. It is used in hair care products, massage oils, and skin care products aimed at combating excessive dryness, preventing signs of aging, and reducing fine lines and wrinkles.

Broccoli seed oil (*Brassica oleracea italica*): This oil contains **antioxidants** and **essential fatty acids** that protect skin against environmental stressors and is intensely hydrating. It is light, nongreasy, noncomedogenic, and easily absorbed. As well as **vitamin C**, it contains **vitamin A**, which helps remove dead skin cells. It's beneficial for all skin types, including sensitive skin. It is used in face creams, face oils, and face serums that target dehydration and the effects of aging.

Bromelain (*Ananas comosus*): Bromelain is an enzyme with anti-inflammatory and antibacterial properties found in the stem or fruit of the pineapple plant. Applied topically, it accelerates the healing of wounds and burns. It also helps remove dead skin cells, restoring health and luster.

Brown sugar: With its natural minerals left intact, brown sugar has all the properties of white sugar with an extra mineral boost that nurtures skin. It is a natural **humectant** and also a natural source of **glycolic acid**. Brown sugar is used in facial and body scrubs, and in bath sugars for soaking as opposed to traditional bath salts. Sugar feeds yeast, however, and can exaggerate breakouts and rashes in some people.

Buriti fruit oil (*Mauritia flexuosa Arecaceae*): Also called aguaje oil, buriti oil is cold-pressed from the wild-harvested fruit of a palm tree native to Brazil. It has one of the highest percentages of **beta-carotene** of any oil and is rich in **essential fatty acids**. It is used in skin care products for its ability to renew cells; protect and repair collagen; increase skin's elasticity, tone, and texture; and reduce and retard signs of aging.

Buttermilk: The **lactic acid** in buttermilk removes dead skin cells, softens, brightens, lightens, moisturizes, and visibly evens skin tone. It contains probiotics that balance skin pH and help maintain healthy skin. Milks are often used in products such as lotions, face creams, bath soaks, and hair care.

Butylated hydroxytoluene (BHT): This synthetic chemical is used in cosmetics as a preservative and **antioxidant**. Studies show it to be both tumor-promoting and anticarcinogenic, depending on the concentration. When applied topically, it affects the liver and kidneys and is associated with toxic effects in lung tissue. The limited studies on its effects on skin show no significant irritation, sensitization, or photosensitization. Some studies claim it is safe for cosmetic use in low concentrations.

Butylparaben: This preservative is used to limit bacterial growth and extend the shelf life of products. Studies suggest that parabens mimic estrogen and can disrupt both male and female reproductive health. The EWG rates it 7/10 on its hazard scale. The FDA has no specific laws for the use of preservatives in cosmetics and claims the lack of reliable evidence/data regarding any harmful effects of parabens on human health suggests no reason to advise against or limit use.

C12-18 acid triglyceride: This synthesized ester of **glycerin** is used as an **emollient** and to enhance the texture and thicken the consistency of lotions and conditioners. The EWG gives it a 1/10 hazard rating, and it's generally regarded as safe for cosmetic use.

Cabbage leaf extract (*Brassica oleracea*): Both the juice and the extract from cabbage leaves are used in skin care for their abundance of minerals and **antioxidants** such as **vitamins C** and **E**. The extract protects against damage, maintains healthy skin cells, and reduces inflammation. Generally used in face creams for acne and wrinkles, its efficacy at reducing inflammation in lactating breasts is being studied.

Cabbage seed oil (*Brassica oleracea*):
Cold-pressed from the seeds, cabbage
seed oil is high in **vitamins C, A, D,** and
K and contains **essential fatty acids.**
This rare and expensive oil is nongreasy
and easily absorbed and is used in small
quantities in face care products rather
than body lotions. It is used to prevent and reverse signs of aging, and to
treat acne.

Caffeine: Caffeine is used topically to
protect skin against UV damage. It has
antioxidant properties and prevents
premature aging. A vasoconstrictor, it is
also used topically to prevent undereye
puffiness and dark circles. The caffeic acid
in caffeine helps skin appear smoother
and is often used in products targeting
cellulite.

Cajeput essential oil (*Melaleuca cajuputi*):
This oil is distilled from the leaves of
a tree related to the tea tree. It has a
strong odor and is generally used in
small amounts in balms and salves for
its antibacterial, antifungal, analgesic,
antiviral, anti-inflammatory, **antioxidant**,
and astringent properties. It is added to
cleansers, massage oils, bath bombs,
and to creams for pain relief and to heal
athlete's foot.

Calcium bentonite clay: This highly absorbent clay generally forms after volcanic
ash ages. It is used for detoxifying and
clearing congested pores and in cosmetics to help them adhere and add natural
water resistance.

Calendula flowers (*Calendula officinalis*):
These vibrant flowers are used in bath
salts, soap, body scrubs, face scrubs, face
masks, and facial steams. They have the
same benefits as **calendula oil** but in a
less concentrated form. The flowers are
dried and either used in powdered form in
face masks and face scrubs, or the petals
are used whole in products such as body
scrubs and facial steams.

Calendula oil (*Calendula officinalis*):
Extracted from calendula flowers into
a carrier oil, this oil is widely used
for its antifungal, antibacterial, and
anti-inflammatory properties. It helps
heal wounds, protects and moisturizes
skin, and reduces redness, making it a
good addition to sunscreens, acne products, salves, face creams, face oils, face
serums, body lotion, and bath soaks. The
soothing oil is suitable for all skin types,
including sensitive and dry skin, and can
be used to treat diaper rash, eczema, and
psoriasis.

California poppy (*Eschscholzia californica*):
Native to California, this species of poppy
contains alkaloids, which are used to fight
wrinkles. There is also an indication that
it helps reduce symptoms of rosacea.
Often used as a calming mild sedative,
it can be added to bath salts.

Camellia oil: Derived from the seeds of
Camellia sinensis, Camellia oleifera, or
Camellia japonica by cold-pressing
or solvent extraction, this oil provides
twice as much **antioxidant** protection as
grape-seed oil, **rose hip oil**, or **vitamin E.**
Packed with high levels of fatty acids,
plus squalene, it increases collagen
production, reduces wrinkles, and is
anti-inflammatory. Additionally, it is
lightweight, quickly absorbed, noncomedogenic, and it soothes sensitive and
irritated skin while increasing skin hydration. Used for dehydrated, mature skin, it
is extremely beneficial in preventing signs
of aging.

**Camphor essential oil (*Cinnamomum cam-
phora*):** Extracted from an evergreen tree
native to Asia, camphor essential oil is

effective in the treatment of acne, inflammation, oily skin, and wound healing. It is concentrated and powerfully scented and is normally used in small amounts for spot treatment.

Camphor hydrosol (*Cinnamomum camphora*): Camphor hydrosol has all the benefits and attributes of the essential oil but in a less caustic form, making it a more versatile way to impart the benefits to skin care products. It is used in acne toners, shampoos and conditioners, and face and body creams. It is also used in eczema and psoriasis sprays and bath products.

Canola oil: Also known as rapeseed oil, canola oil is subject to controversy about its effect on health when taken internally. While there is disagreement among experts on its culinary use, it is showing up more and more in face creams targeting dehydration and aging. It is also used in soapmaking.

Caprylyl caprylate/caprate: This **emollient** and **humectant** is derived from coconut or palm kernel oil. It is mild and generally regarded as safe and suitable for sensitive skin and is often used in body, skin, and baby care products. It leaves skin feeling smooth and dry, and it biodegrades easily.

Capsaicin: Capsaicin is what gives hot peppers their heat. The extract from the pepper is an extremely concentrated analgesic and is used in balms, salves, and creams targeting joint and muscle pain and inflammation. It produces a hot, burning sensation when applied topically.

Caraway essential oil (*Carum carvi*): Produced from caraway seeds, this essential oil has proved effective at treating acne, combating oily skin, healing wounds, and treating infections. It is used in skin care products targeting acne and in salves for wound healing.

Caraway extract (*Carum carvi*): Caraway extract has the same attributes as the ground seeds but is more potent and can be used in a greater variety of products. It can be extracted in water, **glycerin,** or alcohol and is added to face care products to prevent signs of aging, maintain healthy collagen, eliminate dead skin cells, cleanse, and protect against environmental damage.

Caraway seeds (*Carum carvi*): Caraway seeds are ground to a fine powder and used in facial masks and **exfoliants.** They contain **flavonoids,** fatty acids, amino acids, tannins, sugars, and vitamins.

Carotenoid: There are over 600 carotenoids, mainly found in vegetables with yellow, orange, or red flesh. Carotenoids are powerful **antioxidants** often used in skin care products either isolated and synthetic or naturally derived from fruits and vegetables or by using the vegetable itself.

Carrageenan: Derived from red seaweed (**Irish moss**), carrageenan is used as a conditioning, thickening, and **emulsifying** agent in products such as moisturizers, shampoos, and conditioners. Carrageenan increases hydration by holding water onto hair and skin. There are some health concerns about downgraded carrageenan. Only food-grade carrageenan is allowed in cosmetic formulations. In any case, carrageenan molecules are too large for skin to absorb.

Carrot (*Daucus carota*): Carrots are rich in vitamins and nutrients such as **vitamins A, B6,** and K, plus **beta-carotene** and potassium. They protect skin from free radical damage and the deterioration of collagen and leave skin clear, resurfaced, and smooth. Carrots can be used fresh or in a highly concentrated powdered form. The powder is used in face masks and **exfoliants** to treat premature aging, wrinkles, fine lines, and stretch marks. The juice can be used in everything from cleansers to face creams to body lotions.

Carrot root extract (*Daucus carota sativa*): Generally extracted in **glycerin**, this extract is high in **vitamins A** and **E** and **beta-carotene** and is used in face creams, serums, body creams, bar lotions, and lip balms to soothe and soften dehydrated, chapped, flaky, itchy, and uncomfortable skin.

Carrot seed essential oil (*Daucus carota sativa*): This essential oil is antifungal, antibacterial, antiviral, anti-inflammatory, and filled with **antioxidants**. It is used for mature skin, oily skin, eczema, acne, psoriasis, rashes, scars, wrinkles, and wound healing.

Carrot seed oil (*Daucus carota sativa*): Extracted from carrot seed through a cold process, this oil contains a concentrated profile of carotenes and **antioxidants**. It stimulates new cells and tissues, and nourishes, firms, tones, moisturizes, protects, and rejuvenates skin while supplying vital nutrients and **essential fatty acids**. It is noncomedogenic and beneficial for both dry and oily skin, quenching deeply parched skin and helping regulate and balance oil production. Primarily used in antiaging skin care products.

Castor oil (*Ricinus communis*): Often used in soap to increase lather, castor oil is in such demand that many crops are genetically modified to increase yield. The plant itself contains very unhealthy compounds, so careful harvesting and complex processing is necessary. The finished product, however, has no negative side effects. Certified organic castor oil is available. The oil is used for moisturizing, conditioning, and wound healing as it stimulates tissue growth and forms a protective barrier that helps ward off infection.

Catnip (*Nepeta cataria* Linn.): Catnip is a perennial native to Europe, Asia, and Africa. It is most commonly known for its ability to calm, relax, balance, and center. It is a natural astringent and is used to help control dandruff. In skin care it is primarily added to toners and shampoos but is also found in relaxing bath soaks and calming mists.

Cayenne (*Capsicum annuum*): Cayenne is primarily used for muscle pain relief, although it is increasingly used in salves, balms, and lotions for psoriasis and antiaging.

CBD: Cannabinoids (CBD) are one of many compounds in the cannabis plant. CBD has been getting a lot of press about its benefits when taken internally or applied topically. Skin care companies are touting its use for everything from acne to antiaging, but so far there is little research and documentation to substantiate the claims.

Cedar red clay: This powerful detoxifying clay is rich in many natural minerals that help oxygenate skin. Its high absorbency capability and iron content make it extremely beneficial for intense deep pore cleaning and oily skin. Clays work more efficiently when combined with other clays.

Cedarwood essential oil (*Cedrus atlantica*): Also known as Atlas cedar essential oil, this oil is commonly used for its woody scent. Topically, its antiseptic and antifungal properties help treat acne, cellulite, cracked skin, eczema, oily skin, inflammation, and psoriasis.

Cedarwood hydrosol (*Cedrus atlantica*): Cedarwood hydrosol has the benefits of the essential oil but in a less caustic form and can be used undiluted or to replace water in formulations to increase efficacy. It is used in conditioners to control dandruff and in face cleansers, face toners, and face and body creams.

Celery hydrosol (*Apium graveolens*): Celery hydrosol has all the benefits of the extract and essential oil in a less caustic form and can be used undiluted. It is used in facial cleansers and toners targeting aging and acne as well as in pain-relieving sprays.

Celery seed essential oil (*Apium graveolens*): This essential oil is used to balance hormones, invigorate and stimulate cognitive function, ease pain and discomfort, and maintain healthy skin. It is filled with **antioxidants, essential fatty acids**, and anti-inflammatories. It is also used to scent products.

Celery seed extract (*Apium graveolens*): This extract is filled with **antioxidants**, anti-inflammatories, and minerals. Primarily used in skin care creams and lotions, it is now appearing in products targeting muscle aches and pains.

Cellulose acetate: A synthetic compound that comes from cellulose, cellulose acetate can be made into plastics or fabrics. Cellulose is a naturally occurring polymer derived from wood and processed to make cellulose acetate. There are a multitude of modified cellulose polymers used in skin care products for everything from thickening agents and binders to absorbents.

Cellulose acetate microbeads: A bill was passed banning the manufacture and distribution of plastic microbeads due to their detrimental effect on the environment. By July 1, 2018 all products containing plastic microbeads were supposed to be off the market. To replace them as an **exfoliant** that would not cause microdermabrasions, these are one of the newer biodegradable products, which are made from wood pulp from sustainable forests.

Ceteareth-20: This is a blend of cetyl and stearyl alcohols, which are the natural fatty acids in coconut or vegetable oil. It is one of the most common **emollients** used in cosmetic products and also works as an **emulsifier**. It's found in everything from hair dye to sunscreens, cleansers to conditioners. However, the EWG warns of possible contamination with carcinogens such as 1,4-dioxane. This is especially dangerous since ceteareth-20 is a penetration enhancer.

Ceteareth-25: This cleansing and solubilizing agent keeps ingredients evenly dispersed throughout product mixtures. It has more gel-forming and thickening properties than **ceteareth-20** and is used to enhance the texture of products such as lotions, creams, and conditioners. It can be derived from plants, animals, or synthesized in a lab. There is no EWG warning of potential contamination.

Cetearyl alcohol: A viscosity booster and consistency enhancer used to thicken liquid products and increase their foaming capacity, cetearyl alcohol can come from vegetable or **coconut oil** or be synthesized. It is found in many lotions and creams. Because it's a fatty alcohol, it doesn't have the same skin-irritating properties as alcohol, so products labeled "alcohol-free" may still contain cetearyl alcohol. EWG rates it 1/10 on its hazard scale, and it's considered safe for cosmetic use.

Cetyl dimethicone: A synthetic, silicone-based emulsifier that is used as a conditioning agent in many skin and hair care products as well as makeup, particularly primers and liquid foundations. It gives products a creamy, consistent texture, so they go on smoothly while filling fine lines and evening tone. Rated 1/10 on EWG's hazard scale, cetyl dimethicone is considered generally safe for cosmetic use, although there are concerns that because products containing it generally cover the whole face and seal pores, this ingredient disrupts the natural hydration process and possibly creates a dependency on the product, much like petroleum jelly. Because pores are blocked, they're unable to get rid of waste and buildup, which can increase the occurrence of blackheads and breakouts.

Cetyl esters/cetyl palmitate: This is a synthetic wax derived from vegetable or **coconut oil**. It naturally occurs in the head cavities of sperm whales but is now synthesized for cosmetic use. Used in moisturizers and hair care products as an **emollient** and conditioning agent, it gives a smooth, consistent texture and creamy feel. When applied, cetyl esters have no systemic toxicity, sensitization, or photosensitization, and cause little irritation.

Cetyl hydroxyethyl cellulose: Classified as a gum, this compound is used to thicken products and acts as an **emulsion** stabilizer. It helps skin and hair retain moisture while also reducing stickiness. It's often found in moisturizers and conditioners and is generally considered safe for cosmetic use.

Chamomile, German (*Matricaria recutita*): Topically, chamomile calms, soothes, and visibly reduces redness, itching, irritation, and inflammation while keeping skin youthful and glowing. It is also a powerful **antioxidant** used in antiaging products. It is very gentle and suitable for all skin types, even extremely sensitive. Chamomile can be found in many products from soaps to shampoos, face creams to body lotions.

Chamomile, German essential oil (*Matricaria recutita*): This is one of the most widely used essential oils and is found in skin care products for sensitive, dry, aging, and irritated skin. It is often used in spas for relaxation and in bath salts.

Chamomile, German hydrosol (*Matricaria recutita*): Derived through steam distillation of the essential oil, this hydrosol has all the attributes of the flower and essential oil but in a less caustic form that can be used undiluted. It can be used alone as a facial mist or toner or can replace water in any formulation to increase efficacy. It is extremely soothing and calming for both mood and irritated and sensitive skin. It is used in facial toners for sensitive skin and natural baby wipes.

Chardonnay grape seed oil: Grape-seed oil can be made from a variety of grapes, but Chardonnay grape seed oil is limited to the Chardonnay grape. Studies have shown the composition of different grape seeds produce different profiles of the oil. Chardonnay grapes contain **essential fatty acids**, **vitamin E**, and **antioxidants** in amounts significant enough for use in skin care and can be found in face care products, body creams, and body oils targeting the effects of aging.

Chaulmoogra oil (*Hydnocarpus wightianus*): Sometimes called butter, this oil is derived from the seeds of a tropical Indian tree. The oil is extracted by steam distillation, which makes it very pure. It has antiviral and antibacterial properties and is generally used in bars, lotions, salves, or creams targeting psoriasis and eczema, although it can also be found in deodorants and hand sanitizers. It should be used only in small amounts as it is extremely potent and can cause sensitivity.

Cherry blossom extract (*Prunus serrulata*): Cherry blossoms are in the rose family, and both the leaves and petals are edible. The extract, which is made from both, is known for its high levels of **antioxidant**, anti-inflammatory, and skin-lightening properties and **essential fatty acids**. It is very soothing and beneficial for all skin types, helping decongest pores, visibly reduce signs of aging, increase collagen production, and even out skin tone.

Chia seed (*Salvia hispanica*): Edible, nutrient-dense chia seeds come from a flowering plant native to Central America. They contain protein, anti-inflammatories, **antioxidants**, and minerals. The tiny seeds are used whole or ground into powder and added to face masks, facial **exfoliants**, and exfoliating soaps. When water is added to them, they secrete a gelatinous fluid that is soothing, softening, and calming for irritated and sensitive skin.

Chia seed oil (*Salvia hispanica*): Made by pressing and extracting chia seeds, the oil is an intense concentration of the nutrients and benefits of the seeds. It helps prevent free radical damage and rehydrates skin. It also evens out skin tone and texture and reduces redness, scaling, and wrinkles. It is relatively new in the cosmetic world but gaining in popularity.

Chinese ash (*Fraxinus chinensis* Roxb.): This species of flowering tree has been used historically in traditional Chinese medicine and is now appearing in face care products because of its ability to prevent signs of aging and inhibit environmental stress.

Chinese licorice root extract (*Glycyrrhiza uralensis*): This flowering plant native to Asia is a fundamental herb in traditional Chinese medicine. The roots are packed with **flavonoids**, making it an ingredient protective against UV radiation damage. Supremely soothing and moisturizing, with skin tone–evening properties, Chinese licorice is often found in cleansers, toners, moisturizers, and eye creams for sensitive, reddened skin.

Chironji oil (*Buchanania latifolia*): Almond-flavored chironji seeds come from an evergreen tree native to Malaysia, Nepal, and Burma. The seeds are cold-pressed, and the resulting oil is added to antiaging skin care products. The oil is rich in amino acids, **antioxidants**, vitamins, and nutrients that prevent signs of aging, increase cell turnover, and maintain healthy collagen.

Chlorella extract (*Chlorella vulgaris*): Also called dermochlorella, this extract is sourced from green microalgae that typically grow in the waters of Japan and Taiwan. An **antioxidant**, and loaded with amino acids, it protects skin from signs of environmental damage such as pigmentation and sunburn. Some studies show that it promotes collagen production, increases skin firmness, and diminishes the appearance of scars and fine lines. For these reasons, it's found in face masks and antiaging products.

Chloroxylenol: This synthetic liquid antiseptic and disinfectant is primarily found in wound cleaners and antibacterial soaps. It's also used as a preservative and deodorant agent in cosmetic products. At high concentrations, it can cause skin and eye irritation and corrosion and is harmful if swallowed. Currently, studies show no evidence of systemic toxicity in humans and conclude that it's a safe cosmetic ingredient. The EWG, however, rates it 3/10 on its hazard scale.

Chromium hydroxide green: Synthesized from the mineral chromium, this colorant is classified as a "straight color," meaning it isn't mixed or chemically reacted with other substances to create it. Permanently listed by the FDA for cosmetic use, it can be found in makeup, hair dye, nail polish, and bath and skin care products. While allowed in formulations for use around the eyes, it may not be used in products intended for lips. The EWG gives it a hazard rating of 2–4/10.

Chromium oxide greens/chromium(III) oxide: Derived from the mineral chromium, this pigment powder is more stable and permanent than **chromium hydroxide green**. It's classified as a "straight color," meaning it isn't mixed or chemically reacted with any other substances to create it. Permanently listed by the FDA for cosmetic use, it can be found in makeup, hair dye, nail polish, and bath and skin care products. While allowed in formulations for use around the eyes, it may not be used in products intended for lips. The EWG gives it a hazard rating of 2–5/10.

Chrysanthemum: Edible "mums" are cultivated in a variety of colors. Most commonly, people drink tea from white or pale yellow chrysanthemums. Drinking the tea and using the extract helps maintain beautiful skin. Used in creams, it's an anti-inflammatory and helps reduce puffiness.

Cinnamon bark essential oil (*Cinnamomum zeylanicum*): Antiseptic, antibacterial, and antiviral, this oil is used in perfumes and essential oil blends for scenting body products. Some people have a sensitivity to the oil, and it can cause photosensitivity.

Cinnamon bark extract (*Cinnamomum zeylanicum*): This extract has all the attributes of **cinnamon powder** but can be used in a greater variety of products, as it is in either **glycerin** or alcohol. It is often used in products targeting acne but can cause some sensitivity and should be used in very small quantities.

Cinnamon hydrosol (*Cinnamomum zeylanicum*): Cinnamon hydrosol is a beneficial way to get all the attributes of **cinnamon bark** without photosensitivity or skin sensitivity and is used in both antiaging and acne skin care products.

Cinnamon leaf extract (*Cinnamomum zeylanicum*): Cinnamon leaf extract can either be in alcohol or **glycerin**. It is less caustic than the oils and often causes less skin sensitivity. It is used for foot soaks and acne care.

Cinnamon powder (*Cinnamomum zeylanicum*): Made from the inner bark of the tree, cinnamon powder has been used traditionally as a culinary spice and for medicinal purposes. It contains a potent compound, cinnamaldehyde, which is considered responsible for many of its attributes. Cinnamon has **antioxidant**, anti-inflammatory, antibacterial, antiviral, and antifungal properties and helps increase cognitive function. The powder is used in face masks and facial **exfoliants** as well as body and foot scrubs to treat acne and fungus. Caution should be taken when using cinnamon topically as it can cause sensitivity and photosensitivity. It should not be used in bath products.

Citric acid: This is an **alpha hydroxy acid** extracted from citrus fruits. Used for its **antioxidant** and exfoliation properties, citric acid is found in antiaging peels and masks to promote cell renewal and protect against free radical damage. However, **lactic** and **glycolic acids** are believed to be more effective with less likelihood of causing a stinging sensation on skin. Due to its natural acidity, citric acid is also used to adjust the pH of products, preventing them from being too alkaline.

Citronella essential oil (*Cymbopogon nardus*): Extracted from a perennial plant native to tropical parts of Asia, the essential oil has antibacterial, antiseptic, anti-inflammatory, and antifungal properties. It is used as an antidepressant, natural deodorant, and insect repellent. It's a strong essential oil used in very small amounts for oily skin conditions.

Citronella hydrosol (*Cymbopogon nardus*): Citronella hydrosol can be used in more applications than the essential oil and is noncaustic with a milder scent. It is used in acne care, hair care, and in natural insect repellents.

Clary sage (*Salvia sclarea* Linn.): This is a flowering herb native to the northern Mediterranean basin. In skin care, it helps balance sebum production, making it beneficial for both oily and dry complexions. It has powerful antimicrobial properties and contains linalyl acetate, a chemical that works to decrease inflammation and soften scarring.

Clary sage essential oil (*Salvia sclarea* Linn.): This concentrated form of **clary**

sage is used for its aromatherapeutic properties and topically for skin. Added to deodorants, hand sanitizers, acne products, wrinkle treatments, and cellulite products, it is also used in bath soaks. It has a very strong scent that balances and clears the mind. It is generally used in small amounts and should not be used undiluted.

Clary sage extract (*Salvia sclarea* Linn.): This extract is used for alleviating menstrual cramps; controlling oil; treating acne, wrinkles, cellulite, muscle tension, and stress; and for its antimicrobial properties.

Clary sage floral wax (*Salvia sclarea* Linn.): Made from the flower, stem, and leaf, this floral wax is used as a thickening agent and **emulsifier** to add rich, creamy texture and smoothness. It has gentle stimulating properties and is an effective ingredient in detoxifying products.

Clove essential oil (*Syzygium aromaticum*): Clove essential oil contains eugenol, a chemical that may help reduce pain as well as fight infections. It is often used for toothaches as well as in food and beverages. Topically, it is used for its antifungal, antiviral, and antibacterial properties and in the treatment of acne, athlete's foot, cold sores, and wound healing. Its warming, calming scent is added to perfumes and essential oil blends in bath and body care products.

Clove hydrosol (*Syzygium aromaticum*): Clove hydrosol has all the benefits of the essential oil in a noncaustic form and can be used undiluted or to replace water in formulations to increase efficacy and impart aroma. It is used as a mouthwash, for acne skin care, and lotions for athlete's foot and wound healing.

Cocamide DEA (diethanolamine) and MEA (monoethanolamine): These substances are mixtures of fatty acids derived from **coconut oil** or synthesized. Used primarily as thickening, foaming, and emulsifying agents in body washes, shampoos, and conditioners, they are deemed safe for cosmetic use in rinse-off products and in concentrations up to 10% for leave-in products. However, the EWG gives cocamide MEA a 1–4/10 hazard rating and cocamide DEA a 7/10 as a possible human carcinogen. Research shows that when applied topically, there is little toxicity. The vapors, however, are highly toxic, so these ingredients should not be used in aerosol products.

Cocamidopropyl betaine: This synthetic detergent originally derived from **coconut oil** is commonly found in shampoos, makeup removers, body washes, and skin care products. It's believed to cause irritation and/or allergic contact dermatitis and was named Allergen of the Year in 2004. Such reactions could be caused by the ingredient itself or impurities.

Cocoa butter (*Theobroma cacao*): A plant-based fat derived from roasted cocoa beans, cocoa butter is high in **essential fatty acids** and **antioxidants**. Used in lotions and body scrubs, it leaves a nongreasy layer on skin that protects against the elements and locks in moisture. It is readily absorbed and increases skin elasticity and tone as well as prevents stretch marks. While fantastic for skin from the neck down, it should be avoided on the face as it is comedogenic. Most cocoa butter used in cosmetics is decolorized and deodorized to prevent the color and smell in the finished product.

Cocoa leaf extract (*Theobroma cacao*): While cocoa leaves are least known and used, they contain a different profile of antioxidants than the seed extract, making them the perfect complement to the extract to get all the benefits of the cocoa plant in one product. They're used to protect skin against environmental damage and aging, visibly reduce fine lines and wrinkles, and enhance cellular turnover.

Cocoa powder (*Theobroma cacao*): Cocoa powder has all the benefits of the extract in a less concentrated form. It is used for face masks, face **exfoliants**, bath salts and bombs, and in soapmaking and spa treatments.

Cocoa seed extract (*Theobroma cacao*): This extremely concentrated and anti-inflammatory extract is derived from the cocoa bean and is rich in **flavonoids** and **antioxidants**. Topically, it is added to antiaging products to protect skin against environmental damage, reduce fine lines and wrinkles, and increase production of new skin cells and collagen.

Cocodimonium hydroxypropyl hydrolyzed rice protein: This is derived by enzyme, acid, or other means of hydrolysis (the term used when a compound is broken down chemically with the reaction of water). This substance is used in body washes, face cleansers, hair conditioners, and shampoos. While little is known about the long-term effects of this ingredient, it is generally considered safe, although currently the EWG rates it 10/10 for possibly being contaminated with pesticides.

Coconut butter (*Cocos nucifera*): Often confused with **coconut oil** but very different, coconut butter is made by puréeing the coconut meat, including the oil. The resulting butter is solid at temperatures below 76°F and melts at temperatures above. It is high in **essential fatty acids** and vitamins. It also has some antifungal and antibacterial properties, making it a great moisturizer for feet, hands, hair, cuticles, and lips. It can be used alone or in products such as face creams and hand and foot lotions. While many people use it on their face, it can clog pores and is best at under 5% of a cream or 25% of an eye product.

Coconut milk (*Cocos nucifera*): A combination of coconut meat mixed with about 50% water, coconut milk is a natural **emollient** that gently cleans skin without stripping natural oils and provides **vitamins E,** K, **B** complex, and **C,** amino acids, minerals, and **essential fatty acids** vital for skin health but not naturally produced by the body. It combats bacteria and provides intense hydration, and it can visibly reduce the appearance of wrinkles, sagging, and age spots. Very popular, it is used in many products from soap and hair care to face creams and body lotions.

Coconut oil (*Cocos nucifera*): Cold-pressed or expeller-pressed (sometimes called virgin) coconut oil is purer than refined coconut oil. Both are made from the coconut meat, but refined is made from dried meat under high heat that is then bleached, treated with caustic soda, steamed, and filtered. Cold-pressed coconut oil has a strong aroma, so some skin care companies use refined oil to avoid a coconut scent in the finished product. Cold-pressed is generally preferred in skin care products due to the higher level of **antioxidants** and antibacterial properties. Coconut oil increases elasticity, prevents breakouts, and is concentrated with **essential fatty acids**, vitamins, and nutrients vital for skin health.

Coconut water (*Cocos nucifera*): Coconut water is naturally found in young green coconuts. It has less fat and fewer nutrients than coconut milk. It contains **lauric acid**, an antimicrobial. Coconut water is used to impart healthy fluids to keep skin hydrated. It is also used to combat acne, frizzy hair, and athlete's foot.

Coenzyme Q10/Ubiquinone: Also called CoQ10, this is a potent **antioxidant** naturally produced by the body that's vital to proper cell function but decreases with age. The supplement is made in a lab through a yeast fermentation method. When applied topically, the small molecules easily penetrate skin and work by neutralizing harmful free radicals to prevent and repair signs of aging. Because of its skin-rejuvenating properties, it's often used in serums, moisturizers, and other antiaging skin care treatments.

Coffee (*coffea*): Coffee grounds are used in body scrubs for their anticellulite properties, and the caffeine is added to many antiaging and depuffing face care products. Coffee is rich in powerful **antioxidants**; it also aids circulation, is a diuretic, calms irritated and red skin, helps sun-damaged skin and rosacea, and reduces swelling and puffiness around the eyes. It is gentle enough for all skin types, even sensitive.

Coffee butter: This is not a true butter but coffee oil mixed with stearic acid (a naturally occurring fatty acid in plants and animals) to create a viscous buttery texture. Coffee butter has a coffee aroma and is used in cellulite creams, body lotions, body butters, bar lotions, lip balms, and face creams.

Coffee oil: Made by a cold process, coffee oil is a very pure and fairly expensive oil with a coffee aroma. It has the same pH as skin, making it suitable for use on all types of skin. It helps maintain moisture levels and balances oil production, visibly reduces fine lines and wrinkles, and helps in the treatment of acne, cellulite, inflammation, and congested pores.

Collagen protein, hydrolyzed: Collagen proteins are increasingly used in face care products as well as promoted for internal consumption. Bone broth is rich in collagen, and there are many bovine collagen supplements. However, much cosmetic collagen protein comes from other sources such as pigskin, made by an enzymatic hydrolysis process. Topically, collagen is used to increase elasticity and reduce fine lines, sagging, and wrinkles.

Colloidal oats (*Avena sativa L.*): These are made from dehulled oat kernels. They are rich in **polysaccharides**, proteins, lipids, enzymes, **saponins**, **flavonoids**, and vitamins. It is possible to make them at home, but without an industrial machine it isn't possible to grind them as finely as commercial colloidal oats, and they will not be quite as effective. This versatile ingredient can be used to soften and soothe sensitive, itchy, dry skin, rashes, psoriasis, eczema, and acne, and it cleans, exfoliates, and hydrates while also protecting against UV radiation. Most commonly used in bath products, it can also be found in lotions, face masks, and skin care products.

Colloidal silver: Highly popular in skin care as an antibacterial, antifungal, and antiviral for the treatment of acne and as part of a preservation system, the tiny particulates of silver suspended in water are often touted as a skin wonder. However, there is little scientific evidence to support the claims, and the Mayo Clinic considers it unsafe to take internally.

Comfrey root (*Symphytum officinalis*): A perennial herb, comfrey root contains allantoin (gentle moisturizer); rosmarinic (antioxidant), salicylic (helps prevent

blemishes), and caffeic (antiaging) acids; **mucilage** (hydrates and reduces fine lines); **polysaccharides**; and glyco-peptides (antiaging). It is a powerful anti-inflammatory and is used in eye and face creams as well as pain-relieving muscle salves.

Copal essential oil (*Bursera glabrifolia*): This oil, from a tree native to Mexico, is anti-inflammatory and generally used in products for treating acne, although it is also used to heal wounds, treat dermatitis, and condition skin.

Copal extract (*Bursera glabrifolia*): This extract is antibacterial, anti-inflammatory, antiviral, and contains **antioxidants**. It can be used in a wide array of products, mainly face creams and serums, to target acne and aging. It can be used in a higher concentration than the essential oil.

Copal hydrosol (*Bursera glabrifolia*): Copal hydrosol has all the benefits of the essential oil in a less caustic form and can be used undiluted or to replace water in formulations to increase efficacy. It is used in wound-healing sprays and sprays to treat acne, dermatitis, and inflammation.

Copal resin (*Bursera glabrifolia*): This hard, gum-like substance is used to create viscosity and texture in creams and lotions while imparting all the benefits of the oil at less expense. It can also be used in hard bars, lotions, and salves.

Copper peptide: Studies have shown that copper peptide, often considered one of the most powerful skin regeneration ingredients, promotes collagen production, increases skin elasticity, smoothes, tones, tightens, softens, and reduces bumps. It is an **antioxidant** that helps maintain skin's fluid levels and build tissue.

Coriander essential oil (*Coriandrum sativum*): Essential oil made from coriander seeds is used as a blending element in perfumes and essential oil blends for skin and body care. It is also used in natural deodorants, hand sanitizers, and acne products.

Coriander hydrosol (*Coriandrum sativum*): Coriander hydrosol has all the benefits of the essential oil but in a less caustic form, so it can be used undiluted. It is used as a base for natural deodorants, hand sanitizers, and acne toners and cleansers.

Coriander leaf extract (*Coriandrum sativum*): The **antioxidants** in coriander leaf protect against damage and premature aging caused by UV rays. The extract is used in products targeting premature signs of aging and dehydration.

Coriander powder (*Coriandrum sativum*): Coriander powder is made from the seeds. Its **antioxidant** and antibacterial profile makes it suitable for face masks and **exfoliants** for acne. It is becoming extremely popular in natural skin care products as it eliminates the need for preservation systems.

Coriander seed extract (*Coriandrum sativum*): Coriander seeds have a potent **antioxidant** profile and prevent bacteria buildup and the odor caused by it. The extract is often used in acne products and natural deodorants.

Corn silk (maize): Corn silk is the thread-like flexible fibers that grow inside the corn husk. Generally considered a by-product and discarded, it is used in skin care to reduce hyperpigmentation. Studies have shown it to be effective at reducing pigment even on sensitive skin. It is packed with potassium and other vital nutrients, and is anti-inflammatory and an **antioxidant**.

Cornflower (*Centaurea cyanus*): Native to Europe, the blue-purple cornflower petals are often added to products for color. The extract contains anti-inflammatory and **antioxidant** properties and is added to eye care products, foundations, and makeup as well as skin care products for antiaging.

Cornstarch: Cornstarch is made from the corn grain. It is used in cosmetics, baby powder, foundations, makeup, face masks, and deodorant. However, its high percentage of natural sugar encourages the growth of yeast and bacteria, making it contribute to diaper rash, acne, redness, and itching.

Cosmoseuticals: This term, an amalgam of "cosmetics" and "pharmaceuticals," refers to active ingredients that have been researched for their benefits for skin. The FDA does not recognize the term although companies are using it as a marketing aid, creating a new category that they claim is more effective.

Cottonseed oil (*Gossypium herbaceum*): Derived from cotton plants native to sub-Saharan Africa and Arabia, cottonseed oil can be mechanically or chemically extracted. Most commercial cottonseed oil is solvent (chemically) extracted. Rich in fatty acids, it's used for its conditioning effects and can be found in facial serums, eye makeup, and lip balms. It contains gossypol, a crystalline compound that's toxic to livestock and used as a pesticide. It's deemed safe for cosmetic use with established limits on gossypol levels.

Cranberry (*Vaccinium erythrocarpum*): Cranberries, native to North America, are high in **antioxidants**; **vitamins C, A**, and

K; and proanthocyanidins (see **anthocyanins**). Cranberry juice, powder, and extract are all used in skin care to protect against visible signs of sun and environmental damage, discoloration, and fine lines.

Cranberry seed oil (*Vaccinium erythrocarpum*): Cold-press extracted from the seeds, the oil has a unique profile of high **essential fatty acids**, **vitamin E**, and phytosterols (beneficial for hydration and strengthening skin's natural protective barrier). It provides a powerful **antioxidant** blend that helps prevent sun and free radical damage, signs of aging, and dehydration. It can stabilize and extend the shelf life of other, more fragile oils while boosting their antioxidant properties. The oil also aids in the skin's absorption of and ability to use essential fatty acids, plus it tones and tightens.

Cream: Cream is used either fresh or powdered and can replace water in formulations. It gives lotions a silkier, luscious texture as well as imparts **antioxidants**, **essential fatty acids**, and **lactic acid**. Powdered cream is used in powdered masks and **exfoliants** to remove dead skin cells and help keep skin hydrated.

Cubeb oil essential oil (*Piper cubeba*): Extracted from the berries of a pepper plant native to Indonesian islands, this essential oil has antibacterial, antiviral, **antioxidant**, astringent, and analgesic properties and helps detoxify skin and clear congested pores.

Cucumber extract (*Cucumis sativus*): Made from the entire cucumber, the extract contains all the attributes of each part of the cucumber. It is generally extracted in **glycerin** and needs preservation. Knowing the ingredient used to preserve it is important in determining whether the product is acceptable. Research has

shown it can have some skin-lightening, moisturizing, and oil-producing effects. It is used in creams, after-sun products, lotions, cleansers, hair care products, and serums.

Cucumber flesh/juice (*Cucumis sativus*): Primarily composed of water, cucumber is naturally hydrating and visibly reduces redness and inflammation while soothing dry and sensitive skin. It contains **ascorbic acid** and caffeic acid and can help soothe skin irritations and reduce swelling. The juice in the flesh is increasingly found in products aimed at reducing puffiness around eyes and in face creams to replace some of the water in the formulation to increase efficacy.

Cucumber hydrosol (*Cucumis sativus*): Cucumber hydrosol is made through steam distillation of the whole cucumber. The finished product looks like water but has a cucumber aroma. It contains all the attributes of the cucumber and can be used undiluted as a facial mist, toner, or to replace water in any formulation to increase efficacy. It is anti-inflammatory, mildly astringent, and reduces redness and hydrates skin. It is used in facial toners, cleansers, creams, and body lotions.

Cucumber peel (*Cucumis sativus*): Cucumber peel is available powdered and as an extract. It contains a variety of beneficial minerals including silica, which is essential for healthy connective tissue. The peel is cooling and mildly astringent. It is used in face masks, facial toners, and face creams targeting premature aging and blemishes.

Cucumber seed oil (*Cucumis sativus*): Generally only used in face care products, this cold-pressed oil is rich in **vitamin E**, **essential fatty acids**, and **antioxidants**. It is used to combat signs of aging and to treat acne, psoriasis, eczema, sunburn, and redness. It is suitable for all skin types, is noncomedogenic, and is easily absorbed.

Cupuaçu butter (*Theobroma grandiflorum*): Cupuaçu is a pure plant butter from the seeds of an Amazonian rainforest tree. The butter is easily absorbed and filled with **antioxidants**, anti-inflammatories, and **essential fatty acids** that not only protect skin but also heal, soothe, smooth, and soften as well as improve skin's natural moisture barrier to protect it from environmental damage.

***Curculigo orchioides*:** Also known as black musli, this plant, which is rich in **antioxidants** and **bioflavonoids**, is on the verge of extinction, making it a controversial ingredient in skin care. It is used in products for antiaging.

Curcumin: This compound is found in turmeric and has **antioxidant**, anti-inflammatory, antiviral, and antifungal properties. Curcumin will discolor products with an intense yellow if used in a high percentage, making it hard to obtain an active percentage. It can stain skin, so when making products at home, it's best to do a patch test.

Curry plant essential oil (*Helichrysum italicum*): From a plant in the daisy family, this widely used oil is anti-inflammatory, antimicrobial, antiseptic, fungicidal, and an **emollient**. It promotes cell regeneration and is an effective treatment for eczema, psoriasis, wounds, and burns.

Curry plant extract (*Helichrysum italicum*): This extract is used in skin care targeting acne and the effects of aging. It is used topically for skin care and also medicinally.

Curry plant hydrosol (*Helichrysum italicum*): This hydrosol has all the attributes of the essential oil in a less concentrated form and can be used undiluted as a facial toner or mist, or to replace water in formulations to increase efficacy. The hydrosol is used in hand sanitizers, deodorant, and for acne.

Curry plant wax (*Helichrysum italicum*): Curry plant wax is used as a thickening agent and for viscosity and texture. It soothes, moisturizes, softens, and protects skin.

Cyclopentasiloxane: This is a common synthetically manufactured silicone used in many products. It can replace ingredients such as **glycerin** for cost purposes. It's used as a skin conditioner, **emollient**, and lubricant, and for viscosity. Silicone-based products provide waterproofing and add shine, spreadability, and a silky feeling to skin, although they can clog pores.

Cypress essential oil (*Cupressus sempervirens*): From a plant native to the Mediterranean, cypress essential oil has antibacterial, antiviral, and antifungal properties and is often used as part of a preservation system in natural skin care products. It is also used to treat acne, congested pores, cellulite, oily skin, and rosacea; for wound healing; as a natural deodorant; and in perfumes and essential oil blends.

Cypress hydrosol (*Cupressus sempervirens*): Cypress hydrosol has all the properties of the essential oil in a noncaustic form and can be used undiluted or to replace water in a formulation to increase efficacy. It is used as a toner for oily, sensitive, acne- and rosacea-prone skin. It is also added to face cleansers and creams and used as a base in natural deodorants and hand sanitizers.

Cypress leaf extract (*Cupressus semper-virens*): Cypress leaf extract has antiviral, **antioxidant**, and skin-regenerating properties. It does not have the scent of the essential oil, so it can be used in applications where the scent is not desirable. It is used in antiaging and acne products.

Cypress seed oil (*Cupressus sempervirens*): This seed oil is rich in **essential fatty acids**, and research has shown that it absorbs UV rays. It is used to protect skin against environmental damage and dehydration and to prevent and reverse signs of aging.

D&C colors: These are synthetic colors approved for use in cosmetics but not food. (FD&C colors have been approved for both.) While deemed safe for cosmetics, some people find it controversial that these colors cannot be used in food but can be used on skin.

Dandelion (*Taraxacum officinale*): All parts of the dandelion are used. It is high in **vitamins A**, **B** complex, and **C**; and minerals iron, potassium, calcium, magnesium, and zinc. This nutrient profile makes it effective in the treatment of acne and wrinkles. It also aids in hydration and cleansing.

Date extract (*Phoenix dactylifera*): Date extract is an extremely concentrated form of the date's rich nutrient benefits. It is used in high-end antiaging skin care products that target mature skin to visibly reduce signs of aging.

Date paste/powder (*Phoenix dactylifera*): Dates are rich in vitamins, natural fruit sugars, **flavonoids**, **carotenoids**, and phenolic acid (an **antioxidant**). They are anti-inflammatory, gently exfoliate, help clear pores, reduce visible signs of aging, and protect skin from environmental stressors. Both the paste and the powder can be used in many skin care products, from face creams and body scrubs to bath salts and soap.

Date sugar: Date sugar is made by grinding dates without chemical extraction, additives, chemical process, or solvents. The granules, which contain all the nutrients of the date, are very small and dissolve easily in water, so they are used for gentle yet effective facial and body **exfoliants**.

DEA oleth-10 phosphate: A **surfactant** and **emulsifier**, this substance is a compound of diethanolamine and oleic acid (a fatty acid) derived from either plants or animals. It is a controversial ingredient rated 5/10 by the EWG, as it can be cross-contaminated with known carcinogen ethylene oxide and formaldehyde donor 1,4 dioxane; other industry insiders consider it safe.

Dead Sea clay: Located in Jordan and Israel, the Dead Sea contains salt levels 7 to 10 times greater than the ocean, with skin-healing properties that are particularly beneficial for psoriasis. The mineral-rich, soothing clay has a high absorption rate and an ability to profoundly clean pores and minimize their appearance. It tones, lifts, and tightens skin and is used to treat face and body acne, generally in face masks but increasingly in body scrubs, soaps, and bath soaks.

Dead Sea salt: Harvested from the Dead Sea, the salt is prized for its healing attributes. Most sea salts are 90% sodium chloride whereas Dead Sea salt is 10% sodium chloride and has 21 beneficial minerals for skin. It is used to treat acne, psoriasis, eczema, dandruff, and muscle soreness, as well as added to bath soaks to alleviate stress and insomnia.

Decyl glucoside: Considered a mild **surfactant**, this substance is derived from glucose and used in baby shampoo and products for people with sensitive skin.

Decyl oleate: This ingredient is used for its ability to make products nongreasy, slick, and easily applied. It gives skin a very smooth appearance and is used in a variety of products such as color cosmetics, antiaging products, moisturizers, sunscreen, body creams, and face creams. While generally accepted as safe, it is comedogenic and can exacerbate acne and heighten other skin issues such as premature aging.

Deep sea mud/clay: This originated as mud under the sea millions of years ago, making it rich in algae, macro and micro minerals, sodium, and sulfur. Its high concentrations of salt and minerals accelerate natural exfoliation and restore skin's pH. Used as a mild **exfoliant**, it detoxes, reduces cellulite, nourishes, nurtures, and restores lost nutrients. It has a high absorption rate and penetrates deep into pores to adhere to and draw out dirt.

Dehydroacetic acid: This preservative is synthetically derived. Preliminary research on its safety has shown that it's quickly absorbed through the skin and that it is slightly toxic when administered to rats orally. It is deemed safe for use in cosmetics.

Dehydroepiandrosterone (DHEA): Used for mature and aging skin, DHEA increases hydration and moisture levels and is used as a skin brightener, to maintain healthy collagen structure, and to reduce visible signs of aging. It is effective in postmenopausal women as a conditioning agent addressing the significant changes in skin as women age.

Deionized water: Since water can constitute up to 80% of a formulation, the source is critical to the quality of the finished product. City and tap water can contain chlorine and mineral and metal ions that can make **emulsions** difficult and affect the color and purity of the product. Deionized water has had the ions removed, although it can still contain other impurities such as bacteria and viruses. Often, companies will put deionized water through a purification system or systems such as UV light and micron filters.

Delphinindin: This plant pigment can provide protection against oxidative stress, UV damage, and cell damage. It is used in skin care products targeting the prevention and reversal of visible signs of aging such as wrinkles and fine lines.

Denatured alcohol: This is alcohol that has had a denaturant added to render it undrinkable, for use in cosmetics. Denatured alcohol is a controversial ingredient for both its toxicity and skin benefit profiles.

Devil's claw (*Harpagophytum procumbens*): Native to southern Africa, the root of this plant was historically used to heal sores, wounds, and other skin ailments as well as internally to reduce pain and inflammation. Primarily used for its anti-inflammatory benefits in eye serums and creams, it is also gaining popularity for bath soaks.

Dextran: This is a glucose polymer produced by **polysaccharides** and synthesized by bacteria from sucrose. It is used as a thickening agent, to increase moisture levels, to get a smooth creamy consistency, and as an **emollient**. It is also said to have anti-inflammatory and antiaging properties.

Dhupu butter (*Vateria indica*): These seeds from an endangered evergreen tree grown in India have a high percentage of oil that is extracted as butter and used for cooking as well as topically. It is a fairly rare and expensive butter with a very long shelf life. It is used in products for label appeal, stability, and its ability to intensely moisturize.

Diatomaceous earth: This soft powder comes from siliceous sedimentary rock and contains fossilized remains of phytoplankton. It is used to kill insects in gardens and carpet, internally for detoxing, and topically for skin care. It contains high levels of silica. There is little research on any of the claims, but it is said to be antifungal, antibacterial, and antiviral and to decongest pores. It is often used in face masks and **exfoliants**, although because it is said to kill insects by slicing them with its sharp edges, this could potentially cause microdermabrasion when used as an exfoliant.

Diazolidinyl urea: This preservative functions by forming formaldehyde, which means that although the product label may not say formaldehyde, it is in the product. It can be derived from either a plant or animal source. The Contact Dermatitis Institute warns that it may cause a skin reaction when applied.

Dibutylphthalate (DBP, DMP, DEP): These are **phthalates**. Dibutylphthalate (DBP) is a plasticizer used in nail polishes, dimethylphthalate (DMP) is used in hair sprays, and diethylphthalate (DEP) is used as a solvent and fixative in fragrances. In 2010, the FDA claimed that DEP is now the only phthalate still commonly used.

Dicaprylyl carbonate: Used for its skin-conditioning and **emollient** properties, this fat gives a product better spreadability, leaving skin feeling velvety and smooth. It is nongreasy, making it accessible to all skin types. There is little known about whether it is comedogenic. Usually derived from a vegetable source, there is some discussion over whether it is also derived from an animal source.

Dicetyl phosphate: A combination of diesters of cetyl alcohol and phosphoric acid, this ingredient is used as both a **surfactant** and an **emollient**.

Diethanolamine: Studies have confirmed that this substance is carcinogenic in animals although there is inadequate evidence to suggest that it is a possible human carcinogen. It does however cause skin sensitivity and irritation. Metalworking fluids that contain diethanolamine cause a high risk of cancer for workers exposed to it.

Diheptyl succinate: This **emollient** is a natural alternative to silicone, giving the same soft, silky, powdery, light, dry, and nongreasy feel and viscosity. It's both sustainable and biodegradable, however there is little information on whether or not it clogs pores.

Diisostearoyl trimethylolpropane siloxy silicate: This silicone ingredient is used as an **emulsifier** to give a silky, smooth texture to skin. Considered safe for cosmetic use, it does coat and clog pores, which can cause a number of skin issues. It can be derived from an animal source.

Diisostearyl dimer dilinoleate: This is a synthetic ester derived from either plant or animal sources and used as an **emollient** and skin conditioner.

Dill essential oil (*Anethum graveolens*): Extracted from the seeds or leaves and stems of the herb, this oil is used to heal wounds, keep breakouts at bay, and reduce signs of aging.

Dill extract (*Anethum graveolens*): Dill has been used medicinally for hundreds of years for its anti-inflammatory, antibacterial, antifungal, and antiviral properties. Research has shown it to have significant skin penetration, making it a highly potent active ingredient. It helps maintain skin elasticity; decreases breakouts, blackheads, and acne; reduces wrinkles and fine lines; and keeps skin firm and taut.

Dill seed hydrosol (*Anethum graveolens*): This hydrosol has all the benefits of the extract and essential oil and can be used undiluted. It is often used in skin care products such as cleansers and toners to treat acne, or is added to bathwater to reduce skin inflammation, redness, and rashes.

Dimethicone: Also known as polydimethylsiloxane dimethicone, this is a silicon-based polymer. The EWG expresses concerns about organ system toxicity. It is used as an **emollient** in conditioners and skin care products for the glide and smooth, soft, silky feeling it supplies, although it has no skin benefits, is comedogenic, and is contraindicated for overall skin health. Because of its ability to coat skin, it is marketed as an aid to retaining moisture by sealing it in, however it can actually suffocate skin.

Dipotassium phosphate: This is a synthetic, highly water-soluble salt used to adjust pH levels and prevent coagulation in products. There has been little research done on its topical application.

Disodium EDTA: Disodium EDTA is a synthetic preservative, stabilizer, and chelating agent. Chelating agents prevent ingredients in a product from binding with trace elements, such as minerals, often found in tap water. As a result, it's widely used in rinse-off products such as cleansers, shampoos, and conditioners. It's also used in a variety of other formulations to prevent products from deteriorating and to maintain clarity. Studies have shown disodium EDTA to be nontoxic and noncarcinogenic. Some research suggests it may be slightly mutagenic (changes genetic material), but the typical concentration in cosmetic products is too low to cause harm to the human body.

Disodium laureth sulfosuccinate: A mild **surfactant**, this compound is often confused with a sulfate, although it is not. It is often used as an alternative in sulfite-free products such as body washes, bubble baths, and shampoos. Overall, it is considered a more natural alternative since it is biodegradable, but it is made with ethylene oxide, and any ingredient treated with ethylene oxide can become contaminated with 1,4-dioxane, a known carcinogen.

Distilled water: Distilled water is the steam collected from boiled water. This removes salt and most particulates apart from contaminants such as mercury that boil at a lower temperature than water and remain in the steam. It is similar to deionized water, which is generally preferred for skin care, while distilled is acceptable for soapmaking.

DMAE: From the B vitamin choline, this is an **antioxidant** membrane stabilizer. Known for its antiaging and calming effects, it's been widely used for years in skin care formulations such as cleansers, serums, and moisturizers. It's said to help boost collagen production while defending against sagging, thinning skin. The efficacy and safety of DMAE is controversial, though, as some research has shown that DMAE may actually harm or kill skin cells, destroying the mechanisms that naturally keep the skin firm. Its touted antiwrinkle effects may actually be a response to cell damage, which causes the skin to thicken.

DMDM hydantoin: The biggest concern about this ingredient, which is primarily used as a preservation system, is that it's a formaldehyde donor. Such ingredients release low levels of formaldehyde into a product. This means formaldehyde won't be listed on the label but will be in the product. It is used in many products such as baby products, shampoos, conditioners, and "all natural" sulfate-free body washes and shampoos.

Dragonfruit (*Hylocereus undatus*): Also known as pitahaya, this tropical fruit contains highly beneficial **antioxidants** and vitamins that prevent skin oils from becoming rancid, which deteriorates collagen and accelerates skin aging. They also help prevent cell damage and inflammation, as well as protect against UV rays. Dragonfruit is a prebiotic, helping maintain a healthy skin microbiome. The pulp, seeds, and juice are used either fresh or powdered in skin care.

Dragonfruit extract (*Hylocereus undatus*): This extract is made solely from the fruit and is a rich source of **vitamin C** that skin can metabolize and use. Skin care companies use synthetic, common, natural, and fruit sources for vitamin C–enriched products.

Dragonfruit seed oil (*Hylocereus undatus*): Dragonfruit seed oil is prized for its rich and extensive **essential fatty acid** profile as well as **vitamin E**. It is an expensive and rare oil extracted through a cold-press process, making it very pure. A powerful **emollient** that leaves skin softer, supple, and hydrated, it helps maintain healthy collagen, promotes new skin cell production, balances oil production, and visibly reduces signs of aging. It is nongreasy, easily absorbed, noncomedogenic, and suitable for every skin type.

Dulse (*Palmaria palmata*): This red seaweed grows on both the Pacific and Atlantic Ocean coasts. Packed with vitamins and minerals, the dried powder form can be found in face masks and **exfoliants**. It contains a high concentration of polyunsaturated fatty acids that nourish and protect skin's natural oil barrier to keep skin looking firm, plump, and youthful. Due to its high **antioxidant** content, it protects skin by warding off free radical damage.

Dyer's broom extract (*Genista tinctoria*): From a shrub with beautiful yellow flowers, this extract is used as a natural dye for yellow hues and in soapmaking. It is also a rich source of **flavonoids** and used in antiaging face creams.

Egg (ovum): Egg whites contain high levels of collagen, **vitamin A**, and proteins vital for maintaining youthful, healthy skin. They help maintain elasticity, reduce inflammation, minimize the appearance of pores, and make skin look taut, tight, and lifted. There is some controversy about whether or not the collagen in eggs has any transdermal penetration. They are primarily used commercially in face masks and often in a powdered form. When using eggs for skin benefits, it is best to find ones from hens that have not been treated with antibiotics.

Elastin protein, hydrolyzed: This protein generally comes from fish and contains specific proteins found in the connective tissue of the skin and blood vessels. Elastin is important for maintaining youthful skin and is used to revitalize, nurture, moisturize, and visibly reduce the appearance of wrinkles, sagging, and fine lines.

Elderberry fruit extract (*Sambucus nigra*): The most common type of elderberry is native to Europe. Elderberries are packed with powerful **antioxidants** such as **vitamin C**, **flavonoids**, **anthocyanins**, and phenolic acids. Elderberry visibly reduces inflammation, protects skin from environmental stressors and free radical damage, and prevents signs of aging. It has also been shown to fight harmful bacteria, making it beneficial in the treatment of acne.

Elderberry seed oil (*Sambucus nigra*): This oil is used to treat many skin conditions, from acne and psoriasis to burns and inflammation. It has antibacterial, antiviral, antifungal, and anti-inflammatory properties. Studies have shown it accelerates wound healing and the production of collagen. It is used in face creams and oils targeting acne and aging.

Elemi essential oil (*Canarium luzonicum*): Made from the elemi tree's resin, this essential oil is used to balance oil production in mature, dry, or oily skin, and has antibacterial, antifungal, and anti-inflammatory properties. It is often added to face creams and serums.

Elemi extract (*Canarium luzonicum*): Elemi extract can be in either **glycerin** or alcohol and is used for its ability to help tone, tighten, and firm skin. It is antiviral and antibacterial, making it useful for both mature and acne-prone skin.

Elemi resin (*Canarium luzonicum*): Elemi resin has the same scent and attributes of the essential oil but has a solid, gum-like texture and can be added to creams and lotions for texture, viscosity, creaminess, and scent.

Eleuthero (*Eleutherococcus senticosus*): Also known as Siberian ginseng, eleuthero is a deciduous shrub native to the taiga regions of East Asia. Because of possible confusion with *Panax*, or American ginseng, it's currently illegal in the United States to market eleuthero as ginseng. Known for its anti-inflammatory and anti-aging benefits, it firms, tones, and lifts sagging skin. The roots and leaves are rich in vitamins, minerals, and **antioxidants**. Excellent at fighting and protecting against free radical damage, eleuthero also promotes collagen production for supple, youthful-looking skin. It can be found in skin care products for antiaging and eyes.

Emollient: An emollient soothes and softens skin. Emollients can be **essential fatty acids**, oils, or other ingredients that keep skin hydrated and prevent water loss. They differ from moisturizers in that an emollient is just one of the ingredients in a moisturizer.

Emu oil: Made from fat collected from deposits below the bird's skin, emu oil is anti-inflammatory and has some **antioxidant** potential. It is used as a massage oil and in salves for wound healing and pain. Research suggests it increases healthy skin cells and reduces the appearance of wrinkles. Its small particles allow it to effectively penetrate skin. Some people experience sensitivity when using it undiluted.

Emulsifier/emulsion: An emulsifier is an additive that enables two liquids that would not normally mix together (such as oil and water) to form a cohesive and stable substance (an emulsion). In any cosmetic formulation that contains water and oil, an emulsifier is necessary.

Eperua falcata bark extract (*Eperua falcata*): Also known as wallaba, eperua is native to Africa, Brazil, and Venezuela. The bark and resin are anti-inflammatory and **antioxidant**, and contain **bioflavonoids**. The extract is used to treat rosacea, signs of aging, and acne and to prevent damage from environmental stress.

Epigallocatechin gallate (EGCG): This substance in green tea is isolated and used undiluted to boost skin's protective barrier. It increases hydration levels; reduces signs of aging, wrinkles, and fine lines; generates new skin cells and healthy collagen; and protects against free radicals and environmental stress. It is also anti-inflammatory. It's a highly regarded and common ingredient in face care products targeting dehydration, aging, and acne.

Epsom salt: This is not actually salt but a naturally occurring pure mineral compound of magnesium and sulfate. Studies have shown that it has significant transdermal penetration, which led doctors to suggest baths of Epsom salts for patients with magnesium deficiency. It is widely used in products as an **exfoliant**, immune system booster, and foot soak, and for dry skin, acne, and sore muscles.

Essential fatty acids: Essential fatty acids, which are not manufactured by the human body, are required for proper biological function and must be found in the diet. Those found in the epidermis maintain the skin's protective barrier, while those in the dermis help reduce inflammation and prevent collagen damage. Lack of essential fatty acids causes dehydration, premature aging, skin sensitivity, slower wound healing, and scaly skin. A high content of essential fatty acids also helps deliver other nutrients, vitamins, and active ingredients.

Essential oils (see each individual oil for its benefits): Essential oils are made in a steam distillation process that extracts the oil from freshly picked plants. The oils can also be extracted through a chemical process, but those are not considered essential oils. They are used in many skin and body products for their aromatherapeutic properties as well as their active ingredient profile. Using the correct dosage of each essential oil is extremely important, and they should never be used undiluted. Purity of product ranges widely. They also contain volatile organic compounds (VOCs) that can cause dizziness, fatigue, headache, and memory impairment. Currently not much is known about the long-term effects or the safe level of VOCs.

Ester-C: A manufactured combination of **vitamin C** and primarily calcium ascorbate, Ester-C is said to more easily penetrate skin because of its fat solubility. More stable than vitamin C alone, Ester-C is believed to be less vulnerable to environmental exposure breakdown. **Antioxidant**-rich and touted for its anti-inflammatory, elasticity-enhancing, and skin-brightening benefits, it can be found in a wide range of skin care products, including serums and moisturizers.

Esters: Esters are an **emollient** that help smooth skin texture and protect against environmental damage. They are a modified fatty substance made when an organic acid is combined with an alcohol. They don't feel oily when applied, unlike some other emollients, but are highly effective at treating both dry and oily skin.

Ethanol: Ethanol is a type of alcohol produced by fermenting starches such as corn, wheat, and potatoes or sugars such as sugarcane or sweet sorghum with yeasts or through petrochemical processes. When used as a main ingredient in topical products, it can dry out, sensitize, and even erode the skin's surface, accelerating signs of aging. It's often found in toners and wipes, particularly those intended for oily skin due to its astringent, degreasing, and quick-drying nature. It also acts as an antimicrobial, anti-foaming, and viscosity-decreasing agent.

Ethoxydiglycol: This synthetic liquid solvent and carrier is used to thin products and increase penetration of other ingredients. Often used in facial serums, lotions, and shampoos, it also acts as a **humectant**, working to maintain moisture and reduce moisture loss from skin and hair. Studies show that ethoxydiglycol is safe for cosmetic use. It does, however, contain ether, which is associated with issues such as cancer, allergic reactions, and endocrine disruption.

Ethylhexyl olivate: A natural, fatty-acid **emollient** derived from **olive oil,** ethylhexyl olivate can serve as an alternative to silicones to improve the feel and spreadability of products such as creams, lotions, and moisturizers. It prolongs skin hydration, which can increase elasticity for smooth, supple, younger-looking skin.

Ethylhexyl palmitate: Synthesized or derived from plant or animal sources, ethylhexyl palmitate is a mixture of fatty alcohol and palmitic acid. It acts as an **emollient** and texture enhancer to adjust the consistency of products such as moisturizers and lotions. It has a similar feel to silicone and is often used as an alternative. There are no major side effects associated with it, and it's generally regarded as safe for cosmetic use.

Ethylhexylglycerin: This is used primarily as a preservative and is becoming increasingly popular as an alternative to parabens. The EWG gives it a rating of 1/10 although there have been very few studies. Manufacturers claim it to be all natural, and while it does come from a natural source (**glycerin** [glycerol] found in animal fat and vegetable oil), it undergoes many chemical processes.

Ethylparaben: Derived from plants and used as an antifungal preservative in a wide range of products such as lotions, moisturizers, and deodorants, parabens are popular for their gentle efficacy. A study showed a connection between parabens and cancer due to their estrogen-mimicking properties, although the evidence isn't conclusive and parabens are currently deemed safe for cosmetic use in low concentrations.

Eucalyptus essential oil (*Eucalyptus globulus* Labill): Derived from evergreen trees in the myrtle family, this oil is used to boost the immune system, fight infections, calm headaches, repel insects, and for its **antioxidant**, antibacterial, and anti-inflammatory properties. The broad spectrum of properties make it a popular ingredient for many products such as pain salves and bath soaks, deodorants and body lotions.

Eucalyptus hydrosol (*Eucalyptus globulus* Labill): This hydrosol has all the benefits and properties of the essential oil in a noncaustic form that can be used undiluted and to replace water in formulations to increase efficacy. It is highly versatile and used for acne toners, cleansers, natural deodorants, body lotions for pain relief, and calming sprays.

Evening primrose oil (*Oenothera oleum*): Extracted from the seeds of a North American wildflower, this oil is rich in linoleic acid, which is critical for maintaining healthy skin, plus **essential fatty acids**. It has been shown to increase skin's moisture levels, elasticity, and firmness, and to smooth out roughness. It's also an exceptional anti-inflammatory and is beneficial in treating atopic dermatitis.

Exfoliant: An exfoliant is a product or ingredient that removes dead skin cells from the surface of the skin. Physical exfoliators like salt or sugar are used to manually remove dead skin cells, while chemical exfoliators like **alpha hydroxy acid** dissolve the substance that holds cells together.

Fennel bulb extract (*Foeniculum vulgare*): Fennel bulb is rich in amino acids, vitamins, and minerals. The extract is used to reduce inflammation and for overall skin health. It is beneficial for all skin types and protects against environmental damage and premature aging.

Fennel essential oil (*Foeniculum vulgare*): Extracted from fennel seeds, this essential oil is a potent antibacterial with **antioxidant**, antifungal, and anti-inflammatory properties. It is used in perfumes and essential oil blends and topically on mature skin to prevent and reverse wrinkles, and to treat cellulite, congested pores, acne, and oily skin.

Fennel seed hydrosol (*Foeniculum vulgare*): Fennel seed hydrosol has all the benefits of the essential oil in a less caustic form and can be used undiluted or to replace water in formulations to increase efficacy. It is used in cleansers and toners targeting acne and aging skin.

Fennel seed oil, cold-pressed (*Foeniculum vulgare*): The oil is rich in **vitamin C**, potassium, calcium, and iron. It is antibacterial, accelerates skin regeneration, and encourages healthy collagen. It is used in face oils for mature and dehydrated skin as well as in spot treatments for acne.

Fenugreek seed extract (*Trigonella foenum-graecum* L.): From an annual plant native to Asia and Africa, this seed extract provides anti-inflammatory properties and is used to treat eczema, inflammation, and wrinkles. It is used in both skin care and bath soaks.

Feverfew (*Tanacetum parthenium*): A member of the sunflower family native to Europe, feverfew is rich in **antioxidants** and is an anti-inflammatory. In skin care it is used for sensitive skin and to combat rosacea as well as in antiaging products.

Flavonoids: Flavonoids are a large and diverse group of **phytonutrients** found in a wide range of fruits and vegetables. Studies show that flavonoids protect against environmental damage, retard signs of aging, are anti-inflammatory, and help maintain healthy collagen. They are used in both synthetic and natural forms in face creams, face oils, and face serums targeting the prevention and reversal of aging.

Flaxseed oil (*Linum usitatissimum* L.): This oil, generally extracted through a cold process is anti-inflammatory and **emollient**. It has a short shelf life and is sensitive to both heat and light and so should be stored refrigerated in a dark container. Its high concentration of omega-3s and **antioxidants** make it useful topically for dehydration and signs of aging. Ground seeds can be used as a gentle **exfoliant**.

Floral water: While a **hydrosol** is produced through steam distillation, floral waters can be any type of water, from tap to distilled, with the drop of an essential oil or fragrance oil. Companies sometimes call their product a hydrosol when in fact it is a floral water.

Flower essence: A true flower essence is a sun infusion of flowers that are macerated and preserved in brandy. They were developed by Dr. Edward Bach in the 1930s, who said they carry the vibrational imprint of the flower and all of its attributes. They are used medicinally and are becoming an extremely popular topical application in natural skin care.

Formaldehyde: While formaldehyde occurs naturally in everything from cabbage to human bodies, the formaldehyde used in cosmetics is a colorless, flammable, strong-smelling chemical that studies have shown causes cancer in rats and workers exposed to it. There are also many ingredients (e.g., **diazolidinyl urea**) that are formaldehyde donors, which means they release formaldehyde although it is not listed on the product label.

Fragrance: Fragrance encompasses a large category of ingredients used to impart scent to a product. They can also be chemically created to mimic natural essential oils. On a label, fragrance can mean a mixture of synthetic chemicals or a single fragrance. They're taking a lot of heat in the cosmetic industry, especially in the natural sector, because they can contain **phthalates** and other toxic chemicals. Additionally, there's more research coming out about the hazards of breathing in fragrance from candles, air cleansers, and other products that disperse fragrance into the air.

Frangipani absolute (*Plumeria rubra*): Also known as the Hawaiian lei flower, frangipani is native to the tropics. The absolute is expensive but more accessible than **frangipani essential oil**. It is used in perfumes and essential oil blends but is made through solvent extraction as opposed to steam distillation.

Frangipani essential oil (*Plumeria rubra*): Made from frangipani flowers, this extremely expensive and relatively rare essential oil is used in perfumes and some essential oil blends. Beyond its beautiful aroma, it is said to have **antioxidant**, antibacterial, antiviral, and anti-inflammatory properties.

Frangipani extract (*Plumeria rubra*): This extract from the frangipani flowers has **antioxidant** and anti-inflammatory properties and is useful in the treatment of pain and inflammation.

Frangipani hydrosol (*Plumeria rubra*): While hydrosols are generally the most accessible way to get an aroma and the beneficial profile of an ingredient, frangipani hydrosol is rare and expensive. It is used in toners, face creams, and cleansers.

Frankincense (*Boswellia carterii*): There are many types of Boswellia trees that produce essential oils and other ingredients used in cosmetics, but *carterii* is the one most commonly known as frankincense. The extract is anti-inflammatory and used in skin care targeting aging, acne, and psoriasis.

Frankincense essential oil (*Boswellia carterii*): Used in perfumes and essential oil blends for both skin and body care, this oil is very expensive and generally used in small amounts. There is promising research on its effectiveness at killing cancer cells. Topically, it is used in skin care for damaged mature skin, blemishes and blackheads, fungal infections, psoriasis, and to promote cell regeneration.

Frankincense hydrosol (*Boswellia carterii*): This hydrosol has all the attributes of the essential oil in a less caustic form that can be used undiluted or to replace water in formulations to increase efficacy. Extremely versatile, it can be used in toners, bath soaks, foot soaks, and facial sprays to reduce breakouts, repair wrinkles, and heal scars. It also reduces inflammation and helps combat oily skin.

Frankincense resin (*Boswellia carterii*): This hard, gum-like resin can be used in face and body lotions and creams to impart the benefits in the scent and to add viscosity and texture.

French green clay: Also called illite, this clay is used for exfoliation and pore-tightening. The green color comes from decomposed plant material and iron oxide. Good quality clay should be dark green. It is very absorbent and not only draws oils and debris from pores but also pulls blood to the surface of the skin, boosting circulation. It visibly reduces inflammation, tones, and minimizes the appearance of pores.

Gamma linolenic acid (GLA): GLA is a skin-smoothing, unsaturated fatty acid found naturally in **black currant oil/seeds**, **evening primrose oil,** and **borage oil.** It's used in skin care formulations such as moisturizers and creams as an **emollient** and **antioxidant**. It's effective in treating a number of skin conditions, including dermatitis, eczema, dryness, and psoriasis, by preventing water loss. Research suggests that GLA has wound-healing and anti-inflammatory properties, making it beneficial for those with acne.

Garlic essential oil (*Allium sativum*): This essential oil has a strong garlic odor. Garlic is used medicinally for its antibacterial, anti-inflammatory, and antiviral properties. Topically, garlic is generally used to treat acne.

Garlic oil (*Allium sativum*): Garlic oil is an infusion of garlic in a carrier oil. It provides the same benefits as the essential oil but can come in odorless form. DIYers often make and use it to alleviate acne.

Geranium essential oil (*Pelargonium graveolens*): From a perennial shrub native to South Africa and now widely cultivated, this oil is often included in essential oil blends. It has antibacterial properties and is used for eczema, fungal infections, and aging skin.

Geranium essential wax (*Pelargonium graveolens*): Extracted from the flowers, geranium wax is an **emollient** and thickening agent that gives products a creamy feel. It is used in skin care and body lotions for its calming, nurturing effects and astringent properties.

Ginger (*Zingiber officinale*): Ginger is a perennial plant commonly used in culinary applications. It has **antioxidant** and anti-inflammatory properties that protect against free radicals, environmental damage, and signs of aging. It gently draws out toxins, excess oil, and impurities from skin; tones; stimulates; and visibly increases firmness.

Ginger hydrosol (*Zingiber officinale*): Ginger hydrosol has **antioxidants** and anti-inflammatories that can be used undiluted or to replace water in formulations to increase efficacy. It is used in facial cleansers and toners for oily and acne-prone skin.

Ginkgo extract (*Ginkgo biloba*): Native to Asia, ginkgo is thought to be one of the oldest species of tree on Earth. While it has been used internally for some time, topically it is a relatively new ingredient and results are undetermined. It is filled with **antioxidants**, helps balance oil production, and retards signs of aging.

Glacier clay: Traditionally from Canada, glacier clay comes from glacial settlement and is rich in marine compounds, vitamins, and nutrients. It is used to remove toxins and dead skin cells, stimulate circulation, and replenish nutrients.

Glucose oxidase: This synthetic enzyme can also be found naturally in bee pollen and honey. It functions as a skin and hair conditioning agent in products such as creams, lotions, and conditioners. Also used as a stabilizer, it acts as the catalyst in the oxidation of glucose sugar to produce **hydrogen peroxide**.

Glutamine: Glutamine is the most abundant amino acid in the human body and plays a role in more metabolic processes than any other amino acid. Topically, glutamine is valued for its skin-replenishing properties. It is believed to promote youthful-looking skin, and so it is often used in antiaging serums.

Glutathione: This powerful **antioxidant** naturally occurs in the human body, plants, and animals. Research suggests that production gradually decreases with age, which may contribute to visible signs of aging. A combination of three amino acids, glutathione defends against free radical damage, protecting and rejuvenating skin when applied topically. Studies have shown it to improve skin smoothness and reduce wrinkles, making it beneficial in antiaging products such as serums, moisturizers, and masks.

Glycereth-6 laurate: This synthetic ester is essentially the same as **glycereth-26** and is used as a **surfactant** and **emulsifier** in cosmetics.

Glycereth-26/Glycereth-26 phosphate: This is a synthetic ester derived from **glycerin** that comes from animal or vegetable oils. Considered safe for cosmetic use, it is found in body lotions, moisturizers, sunscreens, and hair care products as a skin conditioner, thickener, **humectant**, and foam booster.

Glycerin/glycerol: Glycerin can have either animal or vegetable origins and is a naturally occurring alcohol compound and a part of many lipids. It is a by-product of soap manufacturing. It is used as a humectant, conditioning agent, and solvent to protect skin, as well as for viscosity.

Glycerol monostearate (GMS): This substance is naturally produced by the human body but can be synthesized by reacting **glycerin** with stearic acid (a naturally occurring fatty acid in plants and animals). Considered safe for topical application, it is used as a thickener, lubricant, and **emollient** in cleansers, moisturizers, creams, lotions, and baby products. When used on skin, GMS gives a soft, smooth, nongreasy look and feel.

Glycerol triacetate: Also called triacetin, the primary function of this compound is to prevent microbial growth in products. It's also used as a plasticizer, solvent, and fragrance carrier in hair care, creams, and nail polishes. Considered safe for cosmetic use, glycerol triacetate is also a Generally Recognized as Safe (GRAS) human food ingredient per the FDA.

Glyceryl behenate: This fatty acid acts as a penetration enhancer for other ingredients. It's also an **emollient, surfactant, emulsifier,** and skin-conditioning agent produced synthetically or derived from refined vegetable oils. It is widely used in facial products such as serums, moisturizers, liquid foundations, and lipsticks because it is noncomedogenic. It's considered safe for cosmetic use but the EWG rates it 4/10 on its hazard scale because there's strong evidence that it's an irritant when aerosolized. It should also be noted that its penetration enhancement/increased absorption is favorable only if blended with beneficial ingredients.

Glyceryl cocoate: A **surfactant** made from **glycerin** and coconut fatty acids, this mild, moisturizing, water-soluble **emollient** is used in soaps, body washes, and hair products. Research suggests it may be an irritant, and so it should not be used in aerosols or products intended for use around the eyes. It can also act as a penetration enhancer.

Glyceryl dibehenate: A combination of **glycerin** and the fatty acid **behenic acid,** it's often used as a thickener in cosmetic products such as creams, balms, and concealers. It also serves as an **emollient** and skin conditioner and is rated 1/10 on the EWG's hazard scale.

Glyceryl distearate: This is a compound of **glycerin** and stearic acid (a naturally occurring fatty acid in plants and animals). It's used in skin care formulations such as lotions and creams for its conditioning and **emollient** properties.

Glyceryl esters: These are a large category of ingredients made from **glycerin** and fatty acids. They range from oily liquids to waxy solids and are used in skin and hair care products as **emollients** and lubricants as well as water-binding and thickening agents. They are generally considered safe for cosmetic use in specified concentrations.

Glyceryl myristate: Synthesized from **glycerin** and myristic acid (a fatty acid found in nutmeg, palm oil, **coconut oil,** butterfat, and sperm whale oil), this is generally considered safe for use in cosmetics, with the exception of aerosol products, and can be found in moisturizers, liquid foundations, shaving creams, and hair care as an **emollient** and **surfactant.**

Glyceryl oleate: Made from **glycerin** and oleic acid (a naturally occurring fatty acid found in animal and vegetable fats and oils), it helps **emulsify** ingredients in a formulation. It also functions as an **emollient,** and its pleasant scent makes it popular in fragrance products as well as hair care, makeup, and skin care products.

Glyceryl palmitate: This synthetic **surfactant**, **emulsifier**, and **emollient** is used to thicken products such as creams, lotions, and moisturizers, giving them a smooth, creamy feel. The combination of **glycerin** and palmitic acid (a common saturated fatty acid found in animals, plants, and microorganisms) is considered safe for cosmetic use, though it can be an airborne irritant, so it should not be used in aerosol products.

Glycine soja oil: A natural vegetable oil extracted from soybean seeds, this ingredient contains high concentrations of genistein (a phytoestrogen), **vitamin E**, **essential fatty acids**, and lecithin. A powerful **antioxidant**, when applied topically it can help protect skin by neutralizing free radicals. It's also deeply moisturizing and believed to possess anti-inflammatory and antimicrobial properties. It's a popular ingredient in a variety of skin care products including face and body oils, lip balms, moisturizers, and lotions.

Glycine soja seed extract: This soybean seed extract is a powerful moisturizer when used topically. Full of amino acids, proteins, vitamins, and minerals, it can be found in many products such as soaps, lotions and hair care and skin care products. As an **antioxidant**, it combats free radical damage, reducing the appearance of fine lines and wrinkles while stimulating collagen production, making it a popular ingredient in antiaging skin care formulations.

Glycine soja sterols: Sterols are solid, complex alcohols that lubricate and condition skin and hair. They can come from both plant and animal sources. Glycine soja sterols are derived from the soybean plant and can be found in moisturizers, hair care, and eye creams.

Glycolic acid: This acid has the smallest molecular weight of all the **alpha hydroxy acids** and therefore has significant transdermal penetration. Dermatologists prefer glycolic acid for facial peels. Glycolic acid is also anti-inflammatory and **antioxidant**. It can be naturally derived from sugarcane, but the synthetic form is most common in skin care.

Glycolipids: Glycolipids are fats containing carbohydrates/sugars found naturally in the human body. Often used as a **surfactant** and foam booster, glycolipids are found in products such as shampoos and body washes. Studies suggest that, when applied topically, glycolipids have profound moisturizing effects and improve the barrier function of skin to prevent moisture loss, making them popular in serums and moisturizers for dry skin.

Glycyrrhetinic acid: This active organic compound is isolated from licorice root extract. Known for its anti-inflammatory and skin-soothing properties, it's used in serums, moisturizers, and lotions to restore suppleness to dry, damaged, and/or flaky skin. Studies also suggest that it may encourage cell regeneration in UV-damaged skin.

Goat milk: Goat and cow milk share the same nutritional properties, but goat milk is more easily absorbed by skin. It is gentle enough for all skin types, and packed with **essential fatty acids**, vitamins, nutrients, **antioxidants**, and **lactic acid**. A natural **emollient**, goat milk has an alkaline pH that is perfectly compatible with skin, allowing for quick absorption and hydration. The lactic acid helps remove dead cells from the skin's surface and enhance its natural moisture levels. It's currently very popular in products such as soaps, shampoos, face creams, and body lotions.

Goji berry oil (*Lycium barbarum*): This oil is a highly concentrated source of the active ingredients along with **essential fatty acids**. It is a powerhouse ingredient in antiaging products and suitable for all skin types, as it is noncomedogenic, nongreasy, and easily absorbed.

Goji berry or wolfberry (*Lycium barbarum*): Native to China, goji berries are a super-star **antioxidant** packed with minerals, amino acids, **carotenoids**, and **polysaccharides** that together help firm, tone, and tighten skin. They also protect it from environmental stress, reduce signs of aging, combat wrinkles, increase hydration, brighten skin, and help maintain a healthy glow. Relatively new in skin care, it is primarily used in face care products to prevent and reverse signs of aging.

Gold: Gold is currently hot in the cosmetic industry, with products containing it carrying a hefty price tag and spas offering pricey gold facials. There is no current evidence or research to substantiate the claims of any actual benefits in skin care, and because gold is not soluble, it cannot be absorbed or used by the skin.

Goldenseal (*Hydrastis canadensis*): Native to the United States and Canada, this perennial herb contains **berberine**, which is considered to be antibiotic, anti-bacterial, and antiviral. It is used in skin care to treat acne, in nail oils and foot soaks targeting fungus, and in bath soaks for women's health.

Gooseberry (*Ribes uva-crispa*): This extract contains polyphenol, **flavonoids**, **vitamins A** and **C**, and **anthocyanin**. Studies have shown it to be an antifungal and effective in the treatment of candida. Gooseberries are used to prevent signs of aging, visibly reduce wrinkles and fine lines, and treat acne.

Gotu kola (*Centella asiatica*): Native to Asia and South Africa, this perennial plant is rich in **antioxidants** and **flavonoids** that visibly improve tone and tautness, fight fine lines and wrinkles, reduce signs of aging, boost collagen, and prevent breakouts. Gota kola is currently one of the most sought-after ingredients for antiaging skin care.

Gotu kola oil: (*Centella asiatica*): Also known as brahmi oil, this is not a true oil but gotu kola extract combined with sesame and/or **coconut oil**. It is traditionally used in Ayurvedic medicine for scalp treatment, skin care, soaps, lotions, and to combat stress.

Grape (*Vitis vinifera*): Grape juice without the skin or seeds is a source of **antioxidants**, but it also contains condensed tannins, natural fruit sugars, and **anthocyanins**. These components are highly beneficial when added to facial cleansers, toners, and **exfoliants**. The antioxidant properties protect skin against signs of aging, while the grape pulp and juice help keep pores clean, exfoliate dead skin cells, and resurface and revitalize skin.

Grape alcohol, organic (*Vitis vinifera*): There are many types of alcohol in skin care and all are very different. Made from red wine grapes, organic grape alcohol is extremely expensive, making it an uncommon ingredient. It is used as a preserver, a superhero bacteria-slayer, and an astringent, and it promotes maximum efficacy of all other ingredients. Alcohols in too high concentration can be drying and slightly irritating to sensitive skin.

Grape leaf extract (*Vitis vinifera*): This extract has anti-inflammatory and **antioxidant** benefits as well as being astringent. It is suitable for all skin types and often used in conjunction with other grape extracts to enhance the capabilities of each. It's used in antiaging products, as well as in cleansers and toners.

Grape-seed oil (*Vitis vinifera*): A by-product of winemaking, grape-seed oil comes from pressing the seeds. It is a natural **antioxidant** and contains **alpha-hydroxy acids**, **essential fatty acids**, and other nutrients that make it ideal for aging skin. It also contains anti-inflammatory and antibacterial properties and is noncomedogenic, so it is often used in products targeting breakouts, blemishes, blackheads, and acne. The oil improves skin's elasticity and suppleness, evens skin tone, reduces dehydration, and protects against sun damage.

Grape skin extract (*Vitis vinifera*): The concentration of **antioxidants** in grape skin extract makes it a valuable ingredient in face care and body care products for antiaging. It is also used in soapmaking, where it imparts a lovely light color.

Grape vine extract (*Vitis vinifera*): Grape vine extract is astringent and anti-inflammatory and is used to treat varicose veins. It is generally added to body lotions and creams for smooth, supple, soft, vibrant skin.

Grapefruit essential oil (*Citrus grandis*): This essential oil has a sweet, pungent aroma that is very popular. Studies on its aromatherapeutic effects are generalized and broad; it is said to uplift mood and enhance joy. It is generally used for its aroma and in scent blends in everything from body lotions, bath salts, and shampoo to body wash and body scrubs.

Grapefruit extract (*Citrus grandis*): Extracted from the entire grapefruit in either water or oil, and also available in powdered form, this extract contains **alpha hydroxy acids**, **polysaccharides**, vitamin B6, and **antioxidants**. It is hydrating, helps exfoliate dead skin cells, and is mildly astringent. It is used in body lotions, face creams, face masks, and face serums.

Grapefruit peel extract (*Citrus grandis*): Grapefruit peel is rich in **bioflavonoids**, which makes it advantageous in antiaging products, although it also contains an ingredient that can cause photosensitivity.

Grapefruit seed extract (*Citrus grandis*): Alone, this ingredient is harmless, but it is often contaminated by other ingredients such as **methylparaben**, **triclosan**, and benzethonium chloride. Grapefruit seed extract has been used as a preservation system. Since methylparaben, triclosan, and benzethonium chloride appear in the extract through contamination during processing, they are not listed on the label. Contamination can be an issue with all extracts but is a particular concern with grapefruit seed extract as it tends to get cross-contaminated more than others. Companies now claim their grapefruit seed extract has been tested and is not contaminated. While that answers one issue, what the seed is extracted in is another matter. A common ingredient used for extractions is **propylene glycol**. There are however clean extractions in carriers such as jojoba oil or pure alcohol.

Green tea extract (*Camellia sinensis*): Green, white, and black tea all come from the same plant, the difference being the level of oxidation. Green tea is less oxidized then black and more than white. It contains **antioxidants** and anti-inflammatory polyphenols. Green tea is a powerhouse ingredient used to combat acne as it helps reduce oil production, and to reduce wrinkles in aging skin. Its potent antioxidants visibly reduce signs of aging and protect skin from damage caused by pollutants, free radicals, and UV radiation. It may also help improve the appearance of damaged skin by helping tone and improve elasticity to decrease sagging and fine lines.

Grey salt: Also known as sel gris, this salt is hand harvested from clay-lined salt ponds in the Guérande region of France. This gives it its color as well as a rich supply of minerals. Used in skin care for its high trace mineral content, it is primarily used in products for bathing or exfoliating.

Guaiacwood essential oil (*Guaiacum officinale*): Produced from the wood of a tree native to the Caribbean, this essential oil is used for its firming and tightening effects to help prevent sagging skin and wrinkles. It is also used in perfumes and essential oil blends for scenting skin care, bath, and body products.

Guar gum (*Cyamopsis tetragonoloba*): The guar plant has been cultivated in India and Pakistan for centuries. Guar gum is a thickening and binding agent derived from the endosperm of guar seeds. It functions as a skin and hair conditioner and is used in products such as creams, lotions, and hair care. Studies have shown that it may have anti-inflammatory and wound-healing properties while also extending the shelf life of products.

Guarana seed extract (*Paullinia cupana*): This extract comes from the seeds of the Amazonian guarana plant. It has twice the amount of caffeine as coffee beans. Though more research needs to be done on its topical effects, it's believed to have **antioxidant** and antibacterial properties, protecting skin against damage. Studies have shown that caffeine can help tone and tighten skin, reduce the appearance

of cellulite, and flush toxins. Its powerful anti-inflammatory actions make it a popular ingredient in eye creams and serums where it restricts blood vessels to reduce puffiness.

Guava (*Psidium guajava*): Guava fruits grow on small evergreen trees native to the Caribbean and Central and South America. All parts of the fruit are used both medicinally and topically. The fruit, leaves, and seeds have different benefits. The fruit is filled with **antioxidants**, **flavonoids**, tannins, ascorbic acid, and natural fruit sugars. The pulp is beneficial in cleansing, removing congestion from pores, exfoliating, relieving pain, and in salves for infections. It visibly reduces fine lines and wrinkles and protects skin against environmental damage. The fruit can be used powdered or fresh.

Guava fruit extract (*Psidium guajava*): Packed with **antioxidants**, vitamins, minerals, and nutrients, guava is thought to have skin-protecting properties while toning and brightening skin. Its natural astringent, anti-inflammatory, and antibacterial qualities make it a popular ingredient in a wide variety of skin and hair care products. It's particularly valued in antiaging, acne-fighting, and clarifying formulations.

Guava leaf essential oil (*Psidium guajava*): This essential oil is highly concentrated and has all the benefits of the extract, but it is also used for its aroma. Topically, it is used for athlete's foot and in salves and lotions for pain relief and infections.

Guava leaf extract (*Psidium guajava*): Anti-inflammatory, antiviral, and antibacterial, this extract is effective in the treatment of acne as well as reducing infections and accelerating wound healing. Research suggests it can lighten and brighten skin while protecting against UV and environmental damage. Guava extract is growing in popularity for targeting both acne and aging.

Guava seed oil (*Psidium guajava*): Guava seed oil is cold-pressed without any solvents or chemical extractions, making it a pure and light oil easily absorbed by the skin. It's rich in **lycopene; beta-carotene; vitamins A, B, C, E**, and K; and minerals. It also has antibacterial and antiviral properties. It improves skin texture, decreases sagging, increases elasticity, reverses signs of wrinkles, and combats acne.

Hawthorn berries (*Crataegus species*): A plant in the rose family, hawthorn is rich in **bioflavonoids** and **antioxidants** and is often used in extract form in face care products targeting the effects of aging. It is imperative to know what it is extracted in to determine its efficacy and possible toxicity.

Hazelnut flour (*Corylus avellana*): Also known as a filbert, hazelnuts come from a tree that grows mostly in Turkey, Italy, Spain, and the United States. They contain protein, **B vitamins**, **vitamin E**, magnesium, copper, **essential fatty acids**, and high levels of **antioxidants**. The nuts are finely ground into a flour that is used as a gentle **exfoliant** that also moisturizes, protects, and nurtures skin.

Hazelnut oil (*Corylus avellana*): This cold-pressed oil has the same nutrient content as the nut meat in a more concentrated form. It is noncomedogenic and easily absorbed, making it suitable for all skin types, including sensitive skin. It's a potent moisturizer and contains

antioxidants and mildly astringent tannins, which help to reduce pore size, eliminate bacteria, and decongest pores. This oil increases collagen production and revitalizes skin tone. It is used to reduce wrinkles, fine lines, sun damage, and hyperpigmentation.

Hectorite: Hectorite is a natural white clay derived from a rare, soft mineral. Rich in sodium and magnesium, it is known for its drawing properties, clearing congested pores of impurities and rancid oils. It can be found in a variety of skin care products, particularly masks, and is suitable for both oily and dry complexions as it doesn't dehydrate skin. It's also used as a bulking and suspension agent for products like mineral makeup. It's considered safe for cosmetic use in specified concentrations.

Hematite extract: Derived from the semi-precious stone, hematite extract is high in iron and said to protect, restore, and rebuild collagen. Gemstones may be currently popular in skin care, but there's little substantiating scientific data.

Hemp flour (*Cannabis sativa*): Because the oil content is so high in hempseed, it has to be removed first and then milled into flour. The flour contains all 20 amino acids along with **essential fatty acids**. Amino acids are vital to keeping skin youthful, helping generate new skin cells and protecting collagen. Used as a gentle **exfoliant**, hemp flour removes dead skin cells while it protects, nourishes, and mends.

Hempseed butter (*Cannabis sativa*): This is not a true butter but a combination of hempseed oil and a hydrogenated vegetable oil. The result is a creamy "butter" that has all the attributes of **hempseed oil** in a less concentrated form that can be used in different applications and for different results. Generally it is used to increase the viscosity, richness, creaminess, and texture of a body lotion, body cream, or lotion bar.

Hempseed oil (*Cannabis sativa*): Hempseed oil is a cold-processed and generally unrefined oil. It is highly concentrated and contains all 20 amino acids along with **essential fatty acids**. The oil is noncomedogenic and suitable for all skin types, including sensitive skin. It helps balance the skin's oil production, is anti-inflammatory, and is often used in products for psoriasis, aging, and severely dehydrated skin.

Hexanoyl dipeptide-3 norleucine acetate: Damaged proteins on the skin's surface can obstruct the natural exfoliation process. This synthetic peptide works by competing with these proteins and bolstering the skin's natural shedding ability. Intensely hydrating, it smooths and refines. Research shows that it reduces wrinkles and so is valued for its antiaging properties.

Hexyl laurate: A mixture of hexyl alcohol and lauric acid (a naturally occurring fatty acid), hexyl laurate is used as a skin-conditioning **emollient**, solvent, and thickener. It can be found in sunscreens, foundations, and other makeup and is considered safe for cosmetic use.

Hexyldecanol: A synthetic, nondrying fatty alcohol, this compound is used as an **emollient**, **humectant**, and skin-conditioning agent. It can serve as a base to increase the spreadability of products such as serums, moisturizers, and lotions. Studies have shown that topical application may decrease hyperpigmentation by lightening dark spots and improving skin's overall texture.

Hexylene glycol: This synthetic preservative, solvent and viscosity agent is often used to thin heavy formulations to make them more spreadable. It can be found in products such as body lotions, shampoos, and moisturizers. Although considered safe for use in cosmetic products, some studies suggest that it may be an irritant when applied topically.

Hibiscus flower extract (*rosa-sinensis*): This extract comes from a flowering plant in the mallow family native to tropical areas. The flowers contain high levels of **antioxidants**, **bioflavonoids**, and **vitamin C** that stimulate collagen production, promote tissue regeneration, and help fight signs of aging. It can increase skin circulation, leading to enhanced elasticity and a healthy complexion. It also contains **saponins** and can be used to boost cleansers and facial washes.

Himalayan salt: Mined deep within the Himalayas, this salt is claimed to be one of the purest salts on Earth. The pink color is due to trace minerals like iron. The unique mineral composition makes it beneficial for skin. It is used as a body **exfoliant** and in bath soaks for relaxing, rejuvenating, and replenishing minerals.

Homosalate: A derivative of salicylic acid (see **beta hydroxy acid**), homosalate is found in many chemical sunscreens that protect against UVB radiation. Because it doesn't provide substantial UVA protection, it's combined with other ingredients. It can act as a penetration enhancer. Research shows that homosalate degrades relatively quickly when exposed to sunlight, breaking down into harmful by-products. It may also be a hormone disruptor in both men and women.

Honey (*mel*): This natural **humectant** helps keep skin supple and soft. It is used in products to help eliminate pore buildup, fight acne, heal wounds, reduce scars, and for its antiaging properties. Honey is filled with enzymes, **antioxidants**, and other elements beneficial to skin. It is suitable for all skin types, including sensitive, and can be used undiluted or mixed with other ingredients. DIYers often use honey alone as a wonderful face wash.

Honeybush (*Cyclopia*): The leaves of this South African plant are used for tea. The anti-inflammatory, antifungal, antiviral, antidepressant, and **antioxidant** properties are used for acne and antiaging skin care products as well as bath salts aimed at relaxation.

Honeysuckle extract (*Lonicera japonica*): Made from the flowers, which are dried and then extracted in oil, alcohol, or solvent, this extract contains anti-inflammatory, antiviral, and antibacterial properties and is used to treat acne as well as added to salves for cuts and scrapes. The extract might contain natural **parabens**, and some companies are removing it from their formulations due to bad press about parabens.

Hops essential oil (*Humulus lupulus*): This essential oil is used topically for soothing rashes, irritated skin, redness, itchy skin, and for general skin conditioning.

Hops extract (*Humulus lupulus*): From a perennial plant native to China, this extract has antibacterial, **antioxidant**, anti-inflammatory, and sedative properties. It has been found effective in acne and antiaging products.

Horse chestnut extract (*Aesculus hippocastanum*): Horse chestnuts come from a large deciduous tree native to southeastern Europe. The extract is soothing, anti-inflammatory, and capillary strengthening. It can be found in moisturizers, salves, and toners, particularly those for antiaging.

Horsetail extract (*Equisetum arvense*): The only living genus in its family, horsetail contains more of the trace mineral silicon than any other herb, in a highly absorbable form. Rich in **antioxidants**, vitamins, and nutrients, horsetail is believed to promote a firmer, even-toned complexion that's more resistant to environmental stressors. Also beneficial for dry, sensitive skin, it has powerful moisturizing and anti-inflammatory effects and can be found in products such as cleansers, toners, moisturizers, and shampoos.

Humectant: A substance that promotes the retention of water.

Hyaluronic acid (HA): This acid is naturally produced by the body and helps keep skin youthful, supple, healthy, smooth, and glowing. Production lessens with age. It boosts collagen production and helps skin retain moisture, visually reducing fine lines and wrinkles. HA also helps reduce redness and quickens skin healing. HA is one of the most studied and time-tested ingredients in skin care and is used primarily in face serums.

Hydrogen peroxide: Hydrogen peroxide is a synthetic, liquid chemical compound that's slightly more viscous than water. It's a powerful oxidizer, bleaching agent, and antiseptic with drying properties. Over-the-counter hydrogen peroxide comes in only a 3% concentration due to its potency. Cosmetic use of hydrogen peroxide is controversial. While it's inexpensive, readily available, and generally safe for use on small cuts or scrapes, it's believed to damage skin cells through oxidative stress if used on larger areas. Despite its antimicrobial and drying effects, some studies show that, when applied topically, hydrogen peroxide can lead to increased acne inflammation.

Hydrogenated coco-glycerides: This is a mixture of mono-, di-, and triglycerides derived from hydrogenated **coconut oil**. Hydrogenation allows an oily liquid to remain solid at room temperature, which makes it a useful thickening agent. A skin-conditioning **emollient**, hydrogenated coco-glycerides give skin a soft, smooth appearance and help a product glide onto skin. They can be found in products such as creams, moisturizers, foundations, lipsticks, and eyeliners.

Hydrogenated didecene: This is a skin-conditioning agent derived from the hydrocarbon didecene. Hydrocarbons are organic compounds that contain only carbon and hydrogen (e.g., mineral oil, petroleum, and paraffin wax). It can be found in products such as creams, lotions, hair gels, and foundations. More research needs to be done on the cosmetic safety; although the EWG gives it a hazard rating of 1/10, it's suspected to have nonreproductive organ toxicity.

Hydrogenated lecithin: Lecithin is a natural **emulsifier** and **surfactant** derived from plant and animal sources. Because of its oxidation and instability against heat, cosmetic use of lecithin was limited. Hydrogenated lecithin delivers the same benefits as lecithin with added stability. When applied topically, hydrogenated lecithin soothes, softens, and moisturizes skin. It's often used in products intended for dry and/or mature skin. Although the FDA has rated it GRAS (Generally Recognized As Safe), there are concerns about its penetration-enhancement properties and thus it is considered safe for cosmetic use only in concentrations up to 15%.

Hydrogenated olive oil (*Olea europaea*): Hydrogenated olive oil is made by chemically reacting **olive oil** with hydrogen under high pressure to solidify it for increased stability. Full of **antioxidants** and **essential fatty acids** that are easily absorbed, hydrogenated olive oil is nourishing, moisturizing, and protective to skin. Also known for its soothing and anti-inflammatory effects, it is suitable for sensitive skin and can be found in products like moisturizers, creams, and eye makeup.

Hydrogenated polyisobutene: This synthetic oil is used as a skin-conditioning agent, often as a substitute for mineral oil. It allows for pigment dispersion, particularly in makeup such as lipsticks, eyeshadows, eyeliners, foundations, and concealers. A popular ingredient in waterproof sunscreens, it preserves SPF even after water exposure.

Hydrogenated soybean oil (*Glycine soja/max*): Derived from soybeans and chemically reacted with hydrogen, this oil has a soft, waxy texture that's stable and pleasant to apply to skin. Used as a skin conditioner and thickener, it's commonly found in makeup products such as lipsticks, eyeliners, eyeshadows, blushes, foundations, and concealers, as well as lip balms and moisturizers.

Hydrogenated starch hydrolysate: This substance is made by the hydrogenation of a starch, usually corn, but sometimes potato or wheat. Commonly found in face masks and moisturizers, it acts as a skin conditioner and **humectant**. Studies suggest that it can help calm sensitive skin and reduce irritation.

Hydrogenated vegetable glycerides citrate: This is a mixture of vegetable (often palm) glycerides and **citric acid**

chemically reacted with hydrogen to form a semisolid or solid substance. In cosmetics, it promotes stability while acting as an **emollient** and **emulsifier** and improving texture. It can be found in products such as moisturizers and creams.

Hydrolyzed algae extract: This is made from natural algae that's been broken down by a chemical reaction with water. It contains **polysaccharides** and is used for skin conditioning.

Hydrolyzed keratin protein: This protein can be derived from the hair, feathers, horns, and hooves of various animals. Keratin is rich in amino acids and contains sulfur. It is often used in hair care to strengthen and protect hair but can also be used in facial care products as a protectant.

Hydrolyzed lupine protein: This comes from the seeds of the lupine, which contain all the essential amino acids. It is used in high-end antiaging skin care products to protect against premature aging and reverse visible signs of aging. It is a vegan amino acid ingredient that helps protect collagen and build healthy skin cells.

Hydroquinine: Used as a skin lightener for hyperpigmentation and skin discoloration, hydroquinine was at one point pulled off the market due to safety concerns. The FDA discovered that many products containing it were cross-contaminated with toxins such as mercury. Its safety has been confirmed, and it is available over the counter or at prescription strength from a dermatologist. It generally takes at least four weeks of use to start seeing an effect and many months before the full results are visible.

Hydrosols: Hydrosols are often confused with floral waters, which can be labeled as hydrosols or distillates but are just regular distilled water with a drop of essential oil in it. A true plant hydrosol is the pure distilled water captured during steam distillation. While they look like water, hydrosols have the plant compounds and properties of the essential oils, but in very small amounts, making them gentler and not caustic.

Hydroxyethyl acrylate/sodium acryloyldimethyl taurate copolymer: This is a synthetic polymer that acts as a gelling agent to thicken, stabilize, and opacify products. When used in moisturizers, serums, masks, and sunscreens, it creates a desirable melting sensation when applied that leaves skin feeling smooth and velvety. It is considered safe for use.

Hydroxyethyl urea: Naturally produced by the skin but made synthetically for cosmetic use, this powerful **humectant** helps maintain and replenish the skin's moisture levels. It also stimulates healthy cell turnover, working synergistically with exfoliating ingredients, like **lactic acid**, to slough off dead cells and strengthen the skin's barrier function. It's most commonly found in serums and moisturizers.

Hydroxyethylcellulose: This is a modified, plant-derived amino acid used as a preservative, lubricant, **emulsifier**, thickener, and binder. As a water-soluble substance that can be thickened or thinned, it's used in a wide range of products such as conditioners, mascara, and hair gels. While it doesn't provide any direct benefits to skin or hair, it's a popular cosmetic ingredient due to its versatility.

Hydroxyethylpiperazine ethane sulfonic acid: This substance is often used with ingredients like **glycolic acid** to neutralize pH levels and promote a product's longevity. Studies suggest that when applied topically it can enhance exfoliation and even tone. It can be found in scrubs, serums, and moisturizers. Some preliminary research indicates that in the presence of oxygen it can lead to free radical damage.

Hydroxypropyl cyclodextrin: This is a synthetic or plant-derived **emulsion** stabilizer found in a variety of skin care products, including facial serums and moisturizers. Research suggests that it can enhance the skin-rejuvenating and antiaging properties of other ingredients such as **vitamin C**, retinol, and L-ascorbic acid when used in conjunction with them.

Hydroxypropyl starch phosphate: This synthetic or naturally derived sugar is used as a **surfactant**, texturizer, **emulsifier**, and stabilizer. It can be found in skin care products such as moisturizers. It works to reduce greasiness, giving products a smooth, thick feeling. It's safe for cosmetic use in concentrations up to 10%.

Hyssop essential oil (*Hyssopus officinalis*): This essential oil is antiviral and antibacterial and is used for inflammation, oily skin, eczema, and psoriasis. It is found in face care products for acne and bath soaks for muscle pain.

Hyssop extract (*Hyssopus officinalis*): From an aromatic, semi-evergreen perennial native to southern Eastern Europe, hyssop was traditionally made into tea for respiratory issues and as an antiseptic. The extract can either be in oil or **glycerin** and is generally made from both the leaves and the flowers. It contains antiviral and antibacterial properties and is used in acne cleansers, toners, and face masks.

Hyssop hydrosol (*Hyssopus officinalis*): Hyssop hydrosol has all the benefits of the essential oil in a less caustic form and can be used undiluted or to replace water in any formulation to increase efficacy. It is used in baths for wound healing, eczema, and psoriasis, in body lotions and creams for dehydration, and in toners and cleansers for acne.

I

Illipe butter (*Shorea stenoptera*): This butter is extracted from the nuts of a species of tree that grows in the Southeast Asian jungle. It has a similar profile to cocoa butter and is naturally high in **essential fatty acids**. It can be used undiluted or as part of a formulation. Like cocoa butter, it protects skin and is an excellent moisturizer. It is found in face creams, foundations, body creams, lotion bars, and lip balms, and it is also used in soapmaking.

Imidazolidinyl urea: This synthetic, antimicrobial preservative is often used alongside **parabens**, which release formaldehyde in products. Studies suggest that people exposed to formaldehyde-releasing ingredients may develop a formaldehyde allergy or an allergy to the ingredient itself. Others argue that the amount of formaldehyde released is below the limits for unsafe exposure. One of the most widely used preservatives, imidazolidinyl urea can be found in various products including foundations, shampoos, hair gels, and moisturizers.

Indian barberry (*Berberis aristata*): Also called tree turmeric, barberry is a deciduous evergreen shrub that grows in Europe, Asia, and North America. All parts of the plant are used medicinally for various purposes. The berries are rich in **antioxidants** and the extract is generally used in face care products for antiaging.

Indian barberry bark (*Berberis aristata*): This bark has antiviral and antibacterial properties and protects against cellular damage. It is used in face care products targeting acne and signs of aging.

Indian barberry root (*Berberis aristata*): Topically, this root is used for its antibacterial, anti-inflammatory, and antiviral properties to protect against cellular damage. It is found in skin care products targeting acne to help condition, repair, and combat signs of breakouts.

Indian gooseberry (*Phyllanthus emblica*): These berries from a tree also known as amla contain a potent array of **antioxidants** that have an immediate and long-lasting effect, protecting skin against free radicals and sun damage. They help generate and restore collagen and are used in antiaging skin care products and sunscreens.

Indigo leaf extract (*Indigofera tinctoria*): This extract has **antioxidant**, antiviral, antibacterial, and conditioning properties, making it beneficial for products targeting aging and acne. It is also used as a natural dye in soapmaking.

Inositol: A nutrient in the **vitamin B** complex naturally found in the body tissues of mammals, inositol regulates cell contents and helps them receive hormonal signals, which allows for proper functioning. High levels of inositol in the body can contribute to healthy hair and hair growth; low levels can cause hair loss, dry skin, and eczema. As an ingredient it's synthesized and used in hair and skin care products such as facial serums and shampoos, and in moisturizers as a **humectant**, antistatic, and conditioning agent.

Iodopropynyl butylcarbamate: A synthetic preservative originally used in paints, primers, and coolants to prevent microorganism growth, this preservative is now used in shampoos, conditioners, hair gels, and moisturizers. Evidence suggests it may be toxic to humans and it is linked to gastrointestinal, liver, reproductive, and development issues. However, it's been deemed safe for cosmetic use in concentrations up to 0.1%; concentrations of 0.5% and above may cause skin irritation.

Irish moss (*Chondrus crispus*): Also known as **carrageenan**, Irish moss is actually a seaweed that grows in the Atlantic Ocean. It has high mineral and vitamin levels, and leaves skin silky and smooth. Most often found in hair care as a conditioning agent, it is widely used as a thickening agent and **emulsifier** as well as to soften and hydrate skin. It can be used in creams, lotions, and serums.

Iron oxides: These inorganic chemical compounds have been used as cosmetic pigments since the early 1900s. Though iron oxides can be naturally derived, they're usually synthesized for cosmetic use to ensure purity. They can be found in a wide range of makeup products and bar soaps and are valued for their non-bleeding and moisture-resistant qualities. Applied topically, they are nontoxic and nonirritating.

Isoamyl cocoate: This is a mixture of a natural solvent, isoamyl alcohol, and coconut acid. It may be derived from coconuts or synthesized. A skin-softening **emollient**, it's valued for its light, nonoily, and fast-absorbing feel and can be found in products such as moisturizers, baby lotions, serums, and conditioners, often in place of silicones.

Isoamyl laurate: This ester of isoamyl alcohol and lauric acid is used as a texture enhancer, conditioner, pigment-dispersing agent, and to increase spreadability. It can be plant or synthetically derived and is often used in place of silicones. It is found in products like lotions, moisturizers, and sunscreens.

Isobutyl acetate: This chemical compound is used as a solvent. Though it occurs naturally in raspberries, pears, and other plants, it's usually synthesized for cosmetic use. Found in products such as sunscreens and lip balms, it has a naturally fruity scent at low concentrations.

Isobutylparaben: This is a preservative in the **paraben** family that extends the shelf life of products such as shampoos, conditioners, cleansers, moisturizers, and foundations. Isobutylparaben receives a rating of 8/10 on the EWG's hazard scale. The FDA has no specific laws on the use of preservatives in cosmetics and treats them like any other ingredient. They claim a lack of reliable evidence/data regarding the harmful effects of parabens on human health, and so have no reason to advise against or limit use.

Isoflavonoids: These are a large subclass of **flavonoids**.

Isohexadecane: This is a synthetic cleansing and skin-conditioning agent. Thick and creamy, it's often used to enhance the texture of products but has a dry, powder-like finish. It can be found in moisturizers, sunscreens, serums, makeup removers, and more. The relatively large molecules prevent it from penetrating very deep into skin. Because of this, it's sometimes used to help keep other ingredients, such as **antioxidants**, on the skin's surface.

Isoleucine: This amino acid can be derived from plant proteins such as almonds, cashews, and soybeans. It's believed to promote protein synthesis and is used as a moisturizing and conditioning agent in skin and hair care products. Research also shows that it may be useful in barrier repair, thereby protecting and nourishing skin.

Isononyl isononanoate: A synthetic ester that can be found naturally in cocoa and lavender oils, this substance is used in products such as lipsticks, moisturizers, and foundations as a skin-conditioning **emollient**. Although more research is needed, it has been determined safe for cosmetic use within some limits.

Isopropyl lanolate: This is a chemically modified form of **lanolin**. Popular in makeup formulations, it binds the ingredients of pressed powders. It also functions as a lubricant, giving skin a smooth, glossy appearance. There's some evidence of it being an allergen and/or irritant, though many believe the risk of reaction is low due to the minimal amount used in most products.

Isopropyl myristate: A synthetic oil made from isopropyl alcohol and myristic acid (a fatty acid found naturally in palm oil, **coconut oil,** and butterfat), this is used in products such as creams, lotions, and deodorants to lessen the greasy feel sometimes caused by other ingredients. It also works to fortify skin's natural moisture barrier, thereby keeping skin hydrated. As it is thought to be a penetration enhancer, it's important to pay attention to the other ingredients in a formulation. Some research suggests it may be comedogenic at higher concentrations.

Isopropyl palmitate: A synthetic ester of isopropyl alcohol and palmitic acid, this acts as a conditioner, texturizer, antistatic, and binding agent in many skin and hair care products. It's also believed to enhance skin penetration of other fat-soluble ingredients. Though isopropyl palmitate is safe for cosmetic use and noncomedogenic when diluted, there is evidence that it can irritate skin and/or clog pores if used in higher concentrations.

Isopropyl titanium triisostearate: This synthetic compound is derived from stearic acid, a naturally occurring fatty acid in plants and animals. As an **emollient** and **emulsifier**, it blends well with other ingredients for a nongreasy feel. It is also found in sunscreens to coat titanium dioxide nanoparticles, keeping them suspended and stable.

Isopropyl titanium triisostearate/triethoxy-caprylylsilane crosspolymer: This is a **surfactant** used to control viscosity. It is used in sunscreens and color cosmetics.

Isostearamide DEA: Isostearamide DEA is a synthetic, waxy solid made partly from synthesized fatty acids. Used to boost and stabilize foam, it acts as a cleansing and water-binding agent in foundations, shampoos, and bath products. It's also known to add viscosity to thin, liquid products and act as an antistatic.

Jamaican dogwood (*Piscidia erythrina*): Traditionally used internally for pain, tension, headaches, anxiety, and as a sedative, this deciduous tropical tree is gaining popularity as an ingredient in bath soaks aimed at relaxation. It also contains **antioxidants** and has been making its way into face serums for antiaging.

Jasminum grandiflorum extract: From a plant also known as Spanish jasmine, this extract is used in skin care because of its **antioxidant** content and its natural ability to moisturize, smooth, and even out skin tone. It is suitable for sensitive skin. The extract doesn't have the same scent as the essential oil.

Jasminum grandiflorum essential oil: Extremely popular for its multitude of benefits and its aroma, this essential oil is an antidepressant and antiseptic. It is used to relax muscles, as a calming nerve tonic, to reduce stress, and to rejuvenate, hydrate, and brighten skin. Found in everything from face care to bath soaks, it is one of the most popular scents for perfumes.

Jasminum grandiflorum hydrosol: This hydrosol has all the properties of the essential oil but in a gentle, less concentrated form. It can replace water in formulations to impart the scent and attributes of jasmine.

Jasminum grandiflorum wax: This wax is used as an **emulsifier** to add viscosity and a creamy texture. It has regenerative properties as well as a mild jasmine scent.

Jojoba beads (*Simmondsia chinensis*): Polyethylene beads have long been a popular manual exfoliation method because they do not cause microdermabrasions of the skin. However, there are environmental risks associated with the beads. Jojoba beads are a biodegradable form that avoid the environmental risks but still impart the exfoliation benefits.

Jojoba butter (*Simmondsia chinensis*): There are many cosmetic "butters," none of which are real butter. A true cosmetic butter is made from a single ingredient, such as **mango**, **cocoa**, **shea**, and **babassu**. Most cosmetic butters are an oil such as jojoba mixed with a hydrogenated vegetable oil or stearic acid (a naturally occurring fatty acid in plants and animals). They add a luxurious thickness to creams.

Jojoba oil (*Simmondsia chinensis*): This oil is extracted by cold-pressing the seeds of the jojoba, an evergreen desert shrub. The oil is very similar to skin's sebum, making it noncomedogenic. Filled with **essential fatty acids**, it deeply moisturizes, softens, and conditions dehydrated skin, leaving a breathable protective layer. It is rapidly absorbed, nongreasy, and regulates natural oil production. Also anti-inflammatory, it has positive effects in treating eczema, psoriasis, and acne. Jojoba is one of the most stable oils with a very long shelf life, which makes it an excellent carrier oil. It is costlier than most plant oils and often in short supply.

Jojoba wax: This wax is hydrogenated jojoba oil. It is used in products for slide, as a thickening agent, and to increase solidification. Since it is a natural wax, it is often used as a beeswax replacement in vegan products. Its high **antioxidant** profile helps extend product shelf life. It is eco-friendly, biodegradable, and can be used on sensitive skin. It is extremely nourishing and used in soaps, body butters, lotions, lip balms, hard bar moisturizers, creams, and salves.

Juniper essential oil (*Juniperus virginiana*): Made from juniper leaves, this essential oil is used to reduce cellulite, balance oil production, decongest pores, relieve muscle aches and pain, and treat psoriasis and eczema. Its woody scent is used in essential oil blends for bath and body products and soapmaking.

Juniper hydrosol (*Juniperus virginiana*): Juniper hydrosol has all the benefits of the essential oil in a less caustic form and can be used undiluted or to replace water in formulations to increase efficacy. It is used in body creams and lotions for dehydration, eczema, cellulite, and psoriasis and in facial toners for oily skin and congested pores.

Kacip fatimah (*Labisia pumila*): Native to Malaysia, this small flowering plant has traditionally been used medicinally, especially for women's health issues. It contains both phytoestrogen and phytochemicals. It is primarily used in face creams and serums for mature skin.

Kakadu plum (*Terminalia ferdinandiana*): These plums have been used for thousands of years for medicinal purposes. They're considered to be one of the best sources of **vitamin C**. They also contain antiviral, antifungal, and anti-inflammatory properties and phytochemicals. Beneficial for all skin types, including sensitive, they're often used to treat acne and reduce signs of aging. Quercetin, one of the natural **antioxidants** in the fruit, is highly effective at maintaining healthy skin and reducing wrinkles.

Kalahari melon seed oil (*Citrullus vulgaris*): Also known as wild watermelon, this native African plant is the ancestor of cultivated watermelon. The seed oil is rich in **essential fatty acids** and contains **antioxidants** and **vitamins A**, **C**, and **E**. Light and nongreasy, it is easily absorbed into skin, making it applicable for all skin types. It helps remove excess dirt, oil, and debris from pores. It also helps tighten, firm, and protect skin against environmental damage and retard signs of aging.

Kaolin clay: This gentle clay is suitable for all skin types, including sensitive. It is naturally absorbent, soaks up excess oils, and pulls impurities from pores without causing irritation or redness. White is the most commonly used form, although **yellow**, **red**, and **pink** are also readily available. Each color has different attributes and abilities.

Kapoor katcheri essential oil (*Hedychium spicatum*): Extracted from the rhizomes of a perennial plant, this essential oil is antifungal and antibacterial and primarily used in face oils and face creams to treat acne and in lotions and salves for athlete's foot.

Kefir: This cultured fermented drink tastes similar to **yogurt** but is made using a starter of milk proteins, yeast, and bacteria. While usually made from dairy milk, there are vegan forms available. It is a rich source of **essential fatty acids**, protein, potassium, probiotics, calcium, and **B vitamins** and contains more fat, protein, and probiotics than yogurt. Research has shown kefir to be effective in skin lightening and treating acne.

Kelp (alga): Kelp is a large seaweed in the brown algae family. Among other attributes, kelp is rich in sulfated **polysaccharides**, shown in studies to be effective in protecting skin from UV damage, preventing wrinkles, and gently lightening. It also assists in expelling toxins.

Kiwi flesh/juice (*Actinidia deliciosa*): From a fruiting vine native to China, kiwifruit contain natural enzymes, fruit sugar, **phytonutrients**, **antioxidants**, copper, and potassium. The macerated flesh or juice from the whole fruit (including seeds) is used for its ability to loosen and remove dead skin cells, protect skin from environmental damage, and nurture skin. Generally, it is used in face creams targeting premature aging, fine lines, and wrinkles.

Kiwi seed extract (*Actinidia deliciosa*): Available in both powder and liquid form, the anti-inflammatory, antibacterial, and **antioxidant** properties in this seed extract help maintain skin's natural oil production and decrease acne breakouts. It has been shown to reduce and prevent wrinkles, promote supple skin, and help maintain skin's pH. It is also effective at reducing hyperpigmentation and dark undereye circles, maintaining and increasing moisture levels, and protecting skin from environmental damage.

Kiwi seed oil (*Actinidia deliciosa*): Extracted through a cold process from kiwi seeds, this oil has all the benefits of the seed extract in a highly concentrated form. It also has a potent **essential fatty acid** content, omega-3s, and a high amount of **vitamin E.**

Kojic acid: This acid is made from fungi. It is also a by-product of certain fermented foods such as soy sauce and rice wine. It is used in skin care as a lightening and brightening agent. It also contains some antibacterial and antifungal attributes, making it a positive addition in acne treatment.

Kokum butter (*Garcinia indica*): A true butter, this is extracted from the fruit of the Indian kokum tree and has a fatty acid profile similar to that of **cocoa butter.** It is used in smaller percentages in skin lotions and creams and at higher concentrations in body butters for a rich feel, texture, and hydration. It softens, smoothes, and restores skin's elasticity and moisture content. It is also used in soapmaking.

Kombucha: This is a symbiotic culture of bacteria and yeast grown or cultivated commercially. Commonly thought of as a probiotic health drink, kombucha is making its way into skin care. It protects against environmental and free radical damage, protects collagen, decreases wrinkles, keeps skin soft and supple, evens skin tone, reduces fine lines and wrinkles, and helps keep a healthy bacteria colony that maintains skin's natural acid mantle and overall health.

Kukui nut butter (*Aleurites moluccana*): This is not a pure butter but a combination of kukui nut oil mixed with a hydrogenated vegetable oil to make it feel like a rich creamy butter. It has all the same attributes as the oil, but because of its more solid form it's used differently in formulations, usually to add texture and creaminess to body creams and lotions or hair care products.

Kukui nut oil (*Aleurites moluccana*): Extracted from the seeds of the Hawaiian state tree, this oil has antiviral and antibacterial properties that promote wound healing and collagen production. It is rich in **essential fatty acids**. Generally used in products targeting acne and the effects of aging, it is also added to massage oils and salves for psoriasis, eczema, and stretch marks.

Kundari extract (*Melothria heterophylla*): This root extract is used for its **antioxidant** properties. It protects skin from environmental damage and visibly reduces signs of aging. It is added to face creams targeting the prevention and reversal of aging skin.

L-ascorbic acid (vitamin C): One of the best and most useful forms of vitamin C in skin care, L-ascorbic acid is used as a skin lightening and brightening agent, to prevent and repair damage from sun exposure, for collagen synthesis, and to prevent and minimize fine lines and wrinkles. It is a powerful, highly effective, and widely used **antioxidant**.

Lactic acid: Next to **glycolic acid**, lactic acid is the most popular and researched **alpha hydroxy acid**. Its ability to penetrate the skin is not quite as profound as that of glycolic acid. Different concentrations produce different results. At 2% it begins to hydrate, at 5% it removes dead skin cells, and at up to 10% it provides a more profound and intense exfoliation. It can be derived from dairy milk although the most common forms in skin care are synthetic.

Lanolin: This thick substance, secreted by sebaceous glands in sheep to help keep their coats dry, can be separated into liquid lanolin oil and solid lanolin wax. Lanolin ingredients have excellent moisturizing abilities and are used in a wide range of cosmetic products, including baby and shaving products, as well as skin, hair, and nail care. Some studies have shown lanolin to be an allergen/irritant, while others conclude that there is low risk for reaction because of the negligible amount used in most body care products.

Laureth-4: This is a synthetic polymer composed of lauryl alcohol and polyethylene glycol (**PEG**). A clear, colorless liquid, it's used as an antistatic and **emulsifying** agent in products such as shampoos, conditioners, body washes, foundations, and lipsticks. Although classified as safe for cosmetic use, there is strong evidence that it's an irritant and, due to the presence of PEG, there is also concern about contamination with potentially toxic impurities such as 1,4-dioxane.

Laureth-7: Laureth-7 is a synthetic **surfactant** and **emulsifier** made from chemically modified natural fatty acid, lauric acid, and ethylene oxide. Compared to other laureths, it has relatively low viscosity and can be found in products such as foundations, moisturizers, serums, eye creams, and styling gels. There is some evidence that the lower the numerical value of a laureth, the higher the risk of irritation. There is also concern about contamination with potentially toxic impurities such as 1,4-dioxane.

Laureth-23: A synthetic derivative of **lauryl alcohol**, this is a clear, colorless liquid used as a cleansing and/or solubilizing agent in products such as shampoos, conditioners, hair gels, and shaving creams. Although classified as safe for cosmetic use, more research is needed as there are concerns about contamination, topical irritation, and/or toxicity.

Lauric acid: This is a medium-chain fatty acid abundant in **coconut oil** and also found in palm kernel oil and human, cow, and goat milks. It acts as a **surfactant** in products such as bar soaps, body washes, cleansers, and shampoos. Research suggests it has antimicrobial, antiviral, antibacterial, and moisturizing properties, making it beneficial in combating skin issues from acne to psoriasis to wrinkles. It's considered nontoxic.

Lauroyl lysine: This naturally occurring amino acid is derived from coconut fatty acid. Valued for its skin and hair conditioning properties, it can also be used to enhance the texture of products such as lipsticks, foundations, blushes, eyeshadows, and concealers. It's safe for cosmetic use with limits on concentrations.

Lauryl alcohol: A fatty alcohol that can be synthesized or derived from natural sources such as **coconut oil**, lauryl alcohol is primarily used as an **emulsifier**, stabilizer, and thickener in products such as sunscreens, shampoos, conditioners, and body washes. It has a thick, waxy texture. It is much gentler than other forms of alcohol and can be beneficial to dry complexions as it's nondrying and helps skin retain moisture. That said, some research suggests it may be irritating to especially sensitive skin.

Lauryl glucoside: Used as a dispersant, **surfactant**, and/or foaming agent, this substance is made from coconut or palm oil and sugar often from corn. In products such as shampoos, body washes, cleansers, and hand soaps, it helps water mix with oils and dirt for easy rinsing. Known for its mild nature, it can be found in many baby products.

Lauryl lactate: A combination of **lauryl alcohol** and **lactic acid**, this is found in products such as sunscreens, moisturizers, shampoos, and cleansers for its skin-conditioning and exfoliating effects. Considered safe for cosmetic use, it's also occasionally used as a fragrance ingredient.

Lauryl laurate: A synthetic ester from naturally derived **lauryl alcohol** and **lauric acid** and used for its **emollient** properties and to better integrate other ingredients with the skin's surface, it can be found in products such as sunscreens, conditioners, foundations, and moisturizers. It's considered safe for cosmetic use.

Lauryl PEG-9 polydimethylsiloxyethyl dimethicone: This is a synthetic polymer used as a **humectant**, conditioner, **emulsifier**, stabilizer, and thickener in products like sunscreens, moisturizers, concealers, and foundations. More research is needed as there are concerns about possible toxic contamination.

Lavender (*Lavandula angustifolia or Lavandula officinalis*): A flowering plant in the mint family, lavender is widely cultivated for its beautiful flowers and fragrance. The petals are used in products such as facial steams, scent sachets, and bath salts. Lavender has been shown to calm irritated skin.

Lavender essential oil (*Lavandula angustifolia or Lavandula officinalis*): There are many types of lavender, each carrying its own scent, so many unique essential oils are available. Essential oil, which confers profound aromatherapeutic benefits, is rich in **antioxidants** and anti-inflammatories. It also promotes new cell growth, making it a powerful antiaging ingredient. It's one of the most common essential oils used in every type of skin care product.

Lavender hydrosol (*Lavandula angustifolia or Lavandula officinalis*): Lavender hydrosol has all the properties of the essential oil in a less concentrated form that can be used undiluted. Lavender hydrosol is used in facial toners and mists for acne and oily skin and to replace water in face creams and body lotions to increase efficacy and impart a lovely light scent.

Lavender wax (*Lavandula angustifolia or Lavandula officinalis*): This wax is used as an **emulsifier** and **emollient** for viscosity and rich texture. It is very calming to both skin and mood, making it a perfect wax for sensitive and dehydrated skin.

Lemon balm essential oil (*Melissa officinalis*): This essential oil has some of the same **antioxidant** profiles as the extract, although it is generally used for its aroma to scent lotions, body creams, and soaps, as well as in bath products targeting relaxation and pain relief, body mists for relaxation and insomnia, salves for pain, deodorants, and acne treatments.

Lemon balm extract (*Melissa officinalis*): Lemon balm is a perennial plant in the mint family. Studies have shown it to be effective in the treatment of cold sores, menstrual cramps, headaches, and pain. It contains **antioxidants** and has antibacterial, antiviral, and anti-inflammatory properties. It protects against and reverses wrinkles, fine lines, and signs of aging; helps decrease and combat acne breakouts; and is used in deodorants, foot salves, and calming bath soaks.

Lemon essential oil (*Citrus limon*): Also used aromatherapeutically, lemon essential oil is used topically for its powerful antiviral, antibacterial, astringent, and detoxifying properties that aid in treating acne and deep-cleaning pores. It helps control the overproduction of oil and brightens dull, lackluster, ruddy skin.

Lemon extract (*Citrus limon*): From a mixture of juice and peel or just the peel, lemon extract is much more concentrated and therefore powerful than the peel. It is important to know what the carrier oil of an extract is, as many common carriers are known or suspected to contain toxins. Pure grape alcohol or a plant oil (preferably jojoba due to its stability and long shelf life) are best.

Lemon juice (*Citrus limon*): Lemon is high in **vitamin C**, a commonly used **antioxidant** for skin care. Studies show vitamin C can be effectively absorbed topically. It encourages cell renewal, promotes collagen health, and guards against environmental pollutants and free radicals. Lemon juice is a natural alternative to synthetic vitamin C.

Lemon peel (*Citrus limon*): Lemon peel has much more concentrated levels of **bioflavonoids** and **antioxidants** than the juice, which makes it a powerful alternative. It also contains the essential oil limonene. The combination of juice and peel is often used to get a complete profile. It is used in face care products to prevent damage from environmental stressors, protect collagen, and prevent aging.

Lemon verbena essential oil (*Aloysia citrodora*): Extracted from the leaves and flowers of a plant native to South America, this essential oil is used topically to treat acne and cystic acne as well as to alleviate puffiness and soften skin. It has antibacterial and antiviral properties.

Lemon verbena extract (*Aloysia citrodora*): Generally extracted in alcohol, this can also be extracted in chemical solvents or oil. Depending on the extraction, it may or may not have a gentle aroma. It is less expensive than the essential oil and contains similar properties in a less potent form.

Lemon verbena hydrosol (*Aloysia citrodora*): This hydrosol has the same benefits and properties as the essential oil but in a less caustic form and can be used undiluted or to replace water in formulations to increase efficacy. It is highly beneficial in treating cystic acne and is also used to alleviate puffiness under eyes.

Lemon verbena powder (*Aloysia citrodora*): The powder is more potent than the extract and contains the entire beneficial profile of the essential oil without the strong aroma and in a less caustic form. It is becoming very popular for face masks to treat acne, which can be exacerbated by some chemicals often used to preserve skin care products. This powder is a natural alternative to a preservation system.

Lemongrass essential oil (*Cymbopogon citratus*): This versatile oil is used aromatherapeutically and has antibacterial and antifungal properties that can treat acne and nail fungus. It is found in body sprays, lotions, or soaps to cool the body, and in hand sanitizers and deodorants.

Lemongrass extract (*Cymbopogon citratus*): This herb grows in the tropics, predominantly in Asia. It has **antioxidant**, antifungal, anti-inflammatory, and antibacterial properties. Topically, the extract is used to treat acne, wrinkles, and nail and foot fungus. It is also found in deodorants and hand sanitizers. As with all extracts, it is important to know the carrier, as some carriers are known or suspected to be toxic.

Lemongrass hydrosol (*Cymbopogon citratus*): This is a gentle alternative to the essential oil. It contains the same attributes in a less potent form that can be used undiluted or to replace water in any formulation to add its attributes to facial and body mists to cool an overheated body, natural astringent toners, or for oil and blemish control.

Licorice root extract (*Glycyrrhiza glabra*): Licorice root is a perennial legume native to the Mediterranean and parts of Asia. It's been widely used for centuries as a medicinal herb and is renowned for its soothing, anti-inflammatory and antioxidant benefits. It visibly reduces dark spots, redness, irritation, and inflammation, and protects against environmental stressors, while balancing oil. It gently brightens and moisturizes, helping fade sun damage and treating rosacea and psoriasis.

Lime essential oil (*Citrus aurantifolia*): Lime essential oil is used to treat acne, cellulite, and congested pores, and to heal wounds. It is also added to perfumes and essential oil blends.

Lime extract/flavor (*Citrus aurantifolia*): Lime extract is generally extracted in alcohol but can be in an oil. Used in skin care products to impart scent, the flavored oils are also used in lip balm.

Lime hydrosol (*Citrus aurantifolia*): This hydrosol has all the benefits of the peel and the essential oil and can be used undiluted or to replace water in formulations to impart the attributes and aroma. It is used in acne toners and cleansers.

Lime juice (*Citrus aurantifolia*): Lime juice contains **antioxidants**; **vitamins A, B, C, and D**; calcium; and magnesium. It also contains natural fruit sugar and is anti-inflammatory. Used to protect skin against environmental damage, remove dead skin cells, and keep skin vibrant and healthy, the fresh juice can be added to face creams and lotions, and powder can be added to masks and facial **exfoliants**.

Lime peel (*Citrus aurantifolia*): Lime peel has more **vitamin C** than the juice as well as a higher concentration of **flavonoids**, vitamin B6, magnesium, and potassium. It is anti-inflammatory and used on mature skin to prevent and visibly reduce wrinkles and fine lines. It also helps brighten dull skin and maintain healthy collagen. Powdered peel is added to face masks, face **exfoliants**, and soaps.

Litsea cubeba essential oil: Made from the fruit of an evergreen tree native to China, this essential oil has antibacterial and antiseptic properties that make it useful for oily skin and acne.

Litsea cubeba hydrosol: This hydrosol has all the benefits of the essential oil in a less caustic form that can be used undiluted. It is used for acne toners, acne cleansers, and body lotions targeting acne.

Luffa (*Luffa aegyptiaca*): Also called sponge gourds, luffa are native to Asia. Their fibers are used as a mild **exfoliant** for the body, although they may be too harsh for sensitive facial skin. Often used in spas for body exfoliation, they encourage cellular turnover and healthy skin.

Lutein: This is a naturally occurring **beta-carotene** found in green leafy vegetables such as spinach and kale. A powerful **antioxidant**, it protects skin against environmental stress and damage and is often combined with other antioxidants in skin care products that target premature aging, dehydration, wrinkles, and fine lines.

Lychee extract (*Litchi chinensis*): This extract comes from the lychee fruit and is either in powdered or liquid form. The liquid can be in a base of **glycerin**, solvents, oils, or alcohol. High in **vitamin C** and **antioxidants**, it rejuvenates skin, restores luster, protects against aging, visibly reduces fine lines and wrinkles, and helps skin elasticity.

Lycopene: This bright red carotene gives fruits and vegetables their color. Although its SPF of 3 is not enough to be used as a sunscreen, it does provide some protection against UV radiation. It is used in skin care for premature aging, dehydrated skin, and to prevent and reduce signs of aging. The extract can be found extracted in another plant oil, making it suitable for use in face oils, face creams, and body lotions.

Macadamia nut meal (*Macadamia integrifolia*): The meat of the macadamia nut is milled into a fine powder that has all the benefits of the oil in a less concentrated form. It can be used as a highly effective yet gentle **exfoliant** suitable for all types of skin, including sensitive. It is used in powdered masks, powdered exfoliants, and in spa treatments.

Macadamia oil (*Macadamia integrifolia*): Macadamia oil is extracted through cold-pressing or refinement of the nuts of a tree native to Australia and Hawaii. There is a growing demand for this scarce and expensive oil, which is extremely high in a broad spectrum of **essential fatty acids**, **antioxidants**, amino acids, vitamins, and minerals that help regenerate skin, ward off wrinkles, and combat dehydration.

***Machilus thunbergii* bark:** This tree bark has been used in traditional Chinese medicine but is now showing up in bath salts, body sprays, and aromatherapy products aimed at uplifting and calming mood. It also has some anti-inflammatory properties and can be effective in the treatment and prevention of aging skin.

Madder root (*Rubia tinctorum*): The root of this perennial evergreen is often used as a dye to impart beautiful orange and red hues to textiles. Topically it is used to treat and heal rashes, acne, and wounds.

Magnesium alum silicate: This naturally occurring mineral comes from refined, purified clay. Often used as a thickener, it can be found in shaving creams and lotions, as well as in deodorants for its absorbent properties. Due to its relatively large molecular size, it can't penetrate the skin barrier. It's generally considered safe for use in cosmetics and skin care products.

Magnesium ascorbyl phosphate: A potent **antioxidant** derived from **vitamin C**, this substance is effective at much lower concentrations than vitamin C. It possesses some of the same benefits, such as collagen enrichment. Much less acidic than vitamin C, it can act as a gentler alternative for those with sensitive skin. Known for its anti-inflammatory and brightening/lightening effects, it offers protection against and repair from UV damage, like diminishing the appearance of age spots. It's a popular ingredient in moisturizers and serums.

Magnesium aspartate: An amino acid that supports skin proteins, magnesium aspartate can be animal-derived or created synthetically. Some research shows that when applied topically, it may assist in the delivery of minerals to skin cells, as it does when taken internally. It can be found in skin care products such as moisturizers, serums, and cleansers.

Magnesium carbonate: This mineral salt is often used for its absorbent and pH-balancing qualities in products like foundations, concealers, eyeshadows, and shampoos. Considered safe for use in cosmetics and skin care, it's also used as an opacifying, bulking, and binding agent.

Magnesium laureth sulfate: This is the salt of **sodium laureth sulfate**, commonly found in shampoos as a cleansing agent. Less irritating than other **surfactants** and effective in hard water, it can be used by those with sensitive skin. Though it's classified as a safe ingredient, possible contamination by known toxins ethylene oxide and 1,4-dioxane is a concern.

Magnesium oleth sulfate: This substance is commonly found in shampoos as a cleansing agent. Though it's classified as a safe ingredient, possible contamination by known toxins ethylene oxide and 1,4-dioxane is a concern.

Magnesium sulfate: Also known as Epsom salt, this inorganic salt is found in seawater and mineral deposits. When used topically, it can provide anti-inflammatory benefits, easing muscle soreness and possibly combating acne, which makes it a popular ingredient in bath soaks. Also used as a bulking and conditioning agent, magnesium sulfate can be used in foundations, shampoos, and sunscreens and is deemed safe for cosmetic use.

Magnolia bark (*Magnolia officinalis*): Promoted as one of the new antiaging wonders in skin care, magnolia bark contains very powerful anti-inflammatories that studies show inhibit the activation of NF-KB, a component in the aging processes.

Malachite extract: This extract from the semiprecious stone is used to protect skin. While gemstones may be currently popular in skin care, there's little substantiating scientific data on their effectiveness.

Malic acid (see also alpha hydroxy acid): Malic acid molecules are larger than both **glycolic** and **lactic acid**, resulting in less transdermal penetration and less effective exfoliation. However, it still actively exfoliates and for some people is the best choice as it generally causes less sensitivity. Studies have shown malic acid to

increase collagen production and reverse sun damage and signs of aging. It also may even out pigmentation, fight acne, and reduce wrinkles. It is often made from apples, but for skin care a synthetic form is more commonly used.

Malkangni oil (*Celastrus paniculatus*): Cold-pressed from the seeds of an Indian shrub, this oil is anti-inflammatory, antibacterial, antiviral, and sedative. In skin care it is found in products targeting acne, salves for joint pain and inflammation, and bath soaks for relaxation and stress reduction.

Maltodextrin: Derived from hydrolyzed rice, corn, or potato starch, this sugar is most commonly used as a low-calorie food sweetener. In cosmetics and skin care products such as lipsticks, deodorants, shampoos, moisturizers, and sunscreens, it provides binding and stabilizing properties. Some studies suggest that maltodextrin may enhance the antiaging effects of some weak acids when in the same formulation. Furthermore, it may reduce irritation caused by some acids.

Maltooligosyl glucoside: This is a naturally derived carbohydrate **polysaccharide** combined with a starch that has multiple uses in skin care and cosmetics. It acts as a binding agent, **emulsifier**, hydrator, texture enhancer, and film-forming agent in products such as masks, cleansers, and shampoos. It can replace **glycerin** and is believed to have a soothing effect while giving products a smooth, creamy feel.

Mandarin orange essential oil (*Citrus reticulata*): Extracted from the peel, this essential oil has antiseptic, anti-inflammatory, and astringent properties and is often used for acne.

Mandarin orange hydrosol (*Citrus reticulata*): This hydrosol has all the benefits of the essential oil in a less caustic form. It can be used undiluted or to replace water in any formulation to impart its beautiful scent and attributes. It is also used in bath soaks for rashes and inflammation.

Mandarin orange juice (*Citrus reticulata*): This juice is filled with **vitamins A and C**, calcium, and natural fruit sugars. It removes dead skin cells, helps unclog pores, and protects collagen. The juice can be used fresh or powdered in face masks, cleansers, and creams targeting the effects of aging, and also in body soap.

Mandarin orange peel extract (*Citrus reticulata*): The high levels of **bioflavonoids** and **antioxidants** in Mandarin orange peel are highly effective at preventing wrinkles, sagging, and collagen deterioration. It comes either in an extract or powdered form and is used in skin care aimed at preventing and reversing signs of aging.

Mandelic acid: The least common of all the **alpha hydroxy acids**, mandelic acid has the largest molecules. This means it has the slowest penetration rate and is the best for sensitive skin. Of all the AHAs, it has the most positive effects on skin discoloration.

Mango butter (*Mangifera indica*): Mango butter is extracted from the fruit kernels of a flowering tree native to India. It is a true butter with nothing added to it. Rich in **essential fatty acids**, it is used for body butters, lotions, and creams to add richness, viscosity, and weight. It is extremely moisturizing and beneficial for dehydrated, cracked, brittle, or flaky skin.

Mango fruit (*Mangifera indica*): Mango has antiviral, antibacterial, and anti-inflammatory properties along with natural fruit sugars and **antioxidants**. It gently loosens dead skin cells, helps protect skin, and reduces outbreaks. It can be used either fresh or powdered and is generally found in face masks, cleansers, and exfoliators targeting pore congestion, acne, and aging. Rarely, people can be sensitive to both the peel and fruit.

Mango seed oil (*Mangifera indica*): Mango seed oil is rich in **essential fatty acids**, selenium, copper, zinc, and **antioxidants**. While mango butter is solid at room temperature, the oil is not and can be added to formulations without adding weight and texture, making it perfect for thinner body lotions, body oils, massage oils, and face oils.

Mangosteen fruit juice (*Garcinia mangostana*): This juice has a high concentration of **antioxidants** as well as natural fruit sugars. It is an astringent and is added to face creams and face serums to prevent signs of aging, and to cleansers to gently remove dead skin cells and keep skin soft, supple, and healthy.

Mangosteen seed oil (*Garcinia mangostana*): This oil, pressed from the seeds of a tropical evergreen, is one of the new gold standards in the cosmetic industry. The oil is used in antiaging skin care because of its ability to stabilize cells and retard signs of aging, helping maintain a healthy and youthful appearance. It also helps keep skin hydrated, toned, and tight.

Maple leaf extract: Most people are aware of maple syrup but less so of the leaf extract. Current research suggests it is a potent and powerful ally in preventing and reversing wrinkles and signs of aging. Maple "Botox" is being touted as the hottest new ingredient in antiaging, and companies are rushing to market with products.

Maple syrup: Made from the sap of the maple tree, the syrup is extremely high in natural sugars and **antioxidants**. It also contains magnesium, zinc, iron, and potassium. It gently dissolves and removes dead skin cells, decongests pores, smooths and resurfaces skin, protects against environmental damage, and helps maintain healthy collagen. It is used undiluted in face masks, cleansers, and **exfoliants** as well as added to creams, cleansers, and liquid masks.

Maple water: Maple water is 98% water. It contains a high concentration of calcium, potassium, and magnesium as well as **antioxidants**. It helps maintain proper skin function and is used in face creams for overall skin health.

Marionberry (*Rubus* L.): Due to its **antioxidant** and hydroxy acid content, marionberries are used in early prevention skin care products to resurface skin, remove dead skin cells, decongest pores, protect against environmental damage, and maintain healthy collagen.

Marionberry seed oil (*Rubus* L.): Made by a cold-press extraction, this seed oil is increasingly popular. It is rich in **antioxidants** and effective at protecting against environmental damage. It also maintains healthy collagen and prevents wrinkles and fine lines.

Maritime pine bark extract (*Pinus pinaster*): From a pine tree native to the Mediterranean, this bark extract contains powerful **antioxidant**, anti-inflammatory, antibacterial, antiviral, and pain-relieving properties. It protects against environmental damage, repairs and protects collagen, increases production of **hyaluronic acid**, increases skin's hydration level and elasticity, and visibly reduces signs of aging. It is used in antiaging face creams and serums as well

as in deodorants, hand sanitizers, and acne treatments.

Maritime pine essential oil (*Pinus pinaster*): Distilled from pine needles, this essential oil is antibacterial and antiseptic. It is used in perfumes and essential oil blends as well as in hand sanitizers, deodorants, pain-relieving salves, and acne products.

Marjoram essential oil (*Origanum majorana*): Derived from marjoram flowers and leaves, the essential oil is **antioxidant**, anti-inflammatory, antibacterial, and antifungal and helpful in the treatment of acne and infections.

Marshmallow root (*Althaea officinalis*): Marshmallow is a perennial plant native to parts of Europe, Asia, and Africa and is traditionally used to treat colds, coughs and flu. It has anti-inflammatory and antibacterial properties, and contains **mucilage**, which soothes irritated skin. It is used to treat eczema and acne, and applied topically it helps alleviate pain.

Marula oil (*Sclerocarya birrea*): Made from the pressed kernels of a tree native to South Africa, the profound moisturizing ability of marula oil makes it effective at relieving dehydrated skin, and calming, toning, smoothing, and reducing redness and signs of aging. It has a similar fatty acid profile to **olive oil** and is used in similar applications.

Meadowfoam seed oil (*Limnanthes alba*): This extremely stable oil has a long shelf life and contains powerful **antioxidants** and **essential fatty acids**. It has a very rich feel and leaves skin soft and supple without being comedogenic. It is often used in skin care products as it contains very similar attributes to **jojoba oil** but is less expensive.

Menthol: Either naturally or synthetically derived, this compound found in mint delivers a tingling, cooling effect and is used to relieve joint pain. In small amounts it is added to massage oils for muscle aches and pains. It also promotes better transdermal penetration of other ingredients.

Menthoxypropanediol: This synthetic derivative of **menthol** is used as a cooling, flavoring, fragrance, and fragrance-masking ingredient. A common ingredient in lip-plumping products, it triggers irritation, causing lips to swell. It can also be found in shampoos, conditioners, toners, shaving creams, and aftershaves. Although it receives a 1/10 on EWG's hazard scale, its effects can be up to twice as strong as those of menthol and therefore that much more irritating.

Menthyl anthranilate: This is a synthetic UVA absorber and thus the active ingredient in some sunscreens and SPF lip balms. It's shown to be only moderately effective in protecting against UV radiation and may produce damaging reactive oxygen species when exposed to sunlight. It's not permitted for use in Europe or Japan but is 1 of 17 FDA-approved sunscreen ingredients in the United States.

Menthyl lactate: Used as a cooling fragrance and flavoring ingredient in cosmetics, menthyl lactate is said to be milder and less irritating than **menthol**, but more research is needed. It can be found in many applications such as sunscreens, masks, toners, shampoos, and aftershaves.

Methicone: A silicone-based ingredient found in a variety of products such as foundations, concealers, sunscreens, and moisturizers, methicone creates a protective barrier on skin that slows down water loss to keep skin hydrated. It can also be added to products to make other ingredients either repel or attract water. Due to its large molecular size, methicone doesn't easily penetrate skin, which furthers its protective powers. That said, it can interfere with skin's natural ability to expel waste and toxins and may cause breakouts for those with sensitive and/or acne-prone complexions.

Methyl gluceth-20: Considered a versatile and gentle ingredient that also functions as a foaming and skin-softening agent, this synthetic **emollient** and **humectant** is often used in products such as moisturizers, serums, and cleansers for its ability to retain moisture while opening pores.

Methyl gluceth-20 benzoate: A synthetic ester of **methyl gluceth-20** and benzoic acid, this compound acts as a solvent, **emollient**, and skin conditioner that enhances spreadability of products. It's most commonly found in chemical sunscreens and self-tanning lotions. Although more research is needed, it's considered to have low toxicity and to be safe for cosmetic use.

Methyl glucose sesquistearate: This is a synthetic skin-conditioning agent, **emulsifier**, and **surfactant** made from methyl glucose and stearic acid (a naturally occurring fatty acid in plants and animals). Research shows that it's minimally absorbed by skin, and it has been deemed safe for cosmetic use in its current practices of use and concentration. It can be found in products such as eye creams, moisturizers, and concealers.

Methylchloroisothiazolinone: This widely used synthetic preservative is known for its antibacterial and antifungal properties, although it belongs to a group of chemicals known as isothiazolinones, which are the most potent allergens on the consumer market. There's strong evidence that methylchloroisothiazolinone is an irritant and potential neurotoxin. Because of this, it's primarily found in rinse-off products such as shampoos, conditioners, body washes, hand soaps, and cleansers, though it may be used in leave-on products in concentrations of up to 8%.

Methyldibromo glutaronitrile: This synthetic preservative can be found in products like sunscreens, hand creams, body lotions, facial toners, and cleansers. Research indicates that it's sensitizing when used in leave-on formulations. In Europe, it's banned from use in leave-on products due to a significant rise in allergic reactions. In the United States, it's classified as safe for cosmetic use in low concentrations.

Methylglucoside phosphate: This is a simple sugar derived from glucose that can be found in products such as eye creams, moisturizers, and serums for its skin-softening and antiaging properties. There's evidence that when combined with certain essential amino acids, it can boost skin's collagen and elastin production for improved firmness and elasticity. There are no present concerns regarding its cosmetic safety, though more research is needed.

Methylisothiazolinone: This widely used synthetic preservative and biocide kills and inhibits the growth of microbes. It belongs to a group of chemicals known as isothiazolinones, which are the most potent allergens on the consumer market. There's strong evidence that it's an irritant/allergen and also a suspected neurotoxin. It's approved only for use in low concentrations in rinse-off products such as shampoos, conditioners, body washes, hand soaps, and cleansers.

Methylparaben: This preservative contains **parabens**. It is used to limit bacterial growth and extend the shelf life of products. The EWG rates it 4/10 on its hazard scale. The FDA has no specific laws on use of preservatives in cosmetics and treats them like any other ingredient. They claim a lack of reliable evidence/data regarding the harmful effects of parabens on human health, and so have no reason to advise against or limit use.

Methylpropanediol: An organic, synthetic solvent used in a variety of products, including face masks, moisturizers, eyeliners, toners, and serums, this substance enhances skin absorption of other, active ingredients. No research has shown methylpropanediol to be a toxin or irritant, but it should be used mindfully due to its penetration-boosting effects.

Methylsilanol mannuronate: This organic, seaweed-derived ingredient is used for its skin-conditioning and antistatic properties. When applied topically, it adheres to moisture in the skin to strengthen and firm. It may also help combat the breakdown of collagen and elastin by protecting against free radical damage. Originally used in spa wraps and treatments, it can now be found in products such as moisturizers and serums. There are no known adverse side effects.

Methylsulfonylmethane (MSM): A popular supplement used to boost immune systems, MSM is an organic sulfur compound found naturally in plants and animals and used mostly for joint pain and inflammation. The cosmetic industry claims topical use provides the same benefit profile as a supplement although little research has been done to substantiate the benefits of topical application.

Mexican marigold extract (*Tagetes erecta*): This anti-inflammatory, antiviral, and antibacterial extract is used topically to treat blemishes and blackheads. It is also added to creams and salves for joint pain and inflammation.

Milk (dairy from cows): Although there is controversy over whether digesting cow milk increases breakouts, milk is used topically to prevent them. Milk contains **lactic acid**, **essential fatty acids**, vitamins, enzymes, and proteins. The lactic acid removes dead skin cells, the essential fatty acids replace moisture loss, and the vitamins and proteins help maintain healthy collagen. Avoiding milk from cows that are fed hormones or antibiotics is important for skin care.

Mineral salts: Harvested for over 30 years from an ancient seabed in central Utah, this pure and natural sea salt creates an uninhabitable environment for bacteria. Containing more than 60 trace minerals, the finely milled salt makes a superior bath salt for relaxation and reviving skin. It is also beneficial in deodorants and salt scrub applications.

Moringa leaf extract (*Moringa oleifera*): The extract from the moringa leaf is equally as powerful as the oil. Used for centuries as an antifungal, antiviral, anti-inflammatory, antidepressant, and stress reducer, moringa is a power pack of intense nutrients including proteins, **vitamins A** and **C**, niacin, calcium, potassium, iron, and zinc. It is used topically for its anti-inflammatory and **antioxidant** benefits and its ability to regenerate skin cells.

Moringa oil (*Moringa oleifera*): Cold-pressed from moringa seeds, this oil has a long shelf life and is filled with **antioxidants**, vitamins, and nutrients. It is noncomedogenic, nongreasy, and easily absorbed by skin, evening out skin tone and tightening skin for a youthful, dewy glow. Its anti-inflammatory and collagen-building properties can help diminish the appearance of fine lines and wrinkles while reducing DNA damage in skin cells.

Moroccan chamomile extract (*Ormenis multicaulis*): Moroccan chamomile extract has anti-inflammatory, antifungal, and antiviral properties. It is generally used in skin care to treat acne.

Moroccan chamomile floral wax (*Ormenis multicaulis*): Extracted from chamomile flowers, this wax is used in skin care as an **emollient** and to create viscosity, smooth texture, add thickness, and **emulsify**.

Moroccan red clay (red clay): This clay is naturally high in silica and mineral oxides. Its high iron oxide content gives it a beautiful red color. It is most commonly used to treat rosacea, eczema, and psoriasis as it helps rebalance, calm, and improve skin tone, texture, and elasticity. Its beautiful color makes for use in soapmaking, but it should be cut with other clays when used in face masks or body wraps as it can stain.

Motherwort (*Leonurus cardiaca*): Originally from Europe and Asia, motherwort is a powerful calming herb. Topically, it is used to help heal infections and calm skin. Due to its sleep-inducing, anxiety-relieving attributes it is gaining popularity in aromatherapy and bath soaks.

Mowrah butter (*Bassia latifolia*): Extracted from the fruit of an Indian tree, this butter is pure and without additives. Solid at room temperature, it melts with skin heat and is rapidly absorbed. It is filled with

essential fatty acids, phytochemicals, and potent **antioxidants**. Studies suggest that it may be more effective than **olive oil** at preventing signs of aging. It is generally used in body care such as body creams, butters, lip balms, and hard bar lotions, but it is also found in small percentages in products targeting aging and dehydration.

Mucilage: Mucilage is a viscous substance secreted or extracted from plants. It is used for its ability to visibly reduce fine lines, soothe, soften, hydrate, and help maintain overall skin health. It also helps increase skin's protective barrier and has a plumping effect. It is used to treat rosacea, eczema, and psoriasis and added to antiaging skin care products.

Mung bean (*Vigna radiata*): Mung beans are an edible legume used in skin care as gentle and mild **exfoliants**. They help maintain and even out skin tone and texture for a healthy glow.

Mungongo oil (*Schinziophyton rautanenii*): The oil is extracted from the nuts of a tree native to Africa. It contains amino acids, minerals, **vitamin E**, and **essential fatty acids**, making it a superstar ingredient for skin care. It is often added to face care products targeting the effects of aging but is also found in lip balms, body lotions, oils, and butters. It is suitable for all types of skin, including sensitive.

Mushrooms: A type of fungus that grows in moist areas worldwide, mushrooms are rich in **vitamin D**, selenium, and **antioxidants**. They are used in skin care to reduce inflammation and irritation and soothe even the most sensitive skin, as well as for skin brightening and lightening, and to repair, reduce, and protect against aging and wrinkles. The extract is used in many products including soaps, face creams, serums, and shampoos.

Muskmelon seed oil (*Cucumis melo var. cantalupensis*): Also known as cantaloupe seed oil, this oil is extracted by cold-pressing cantaloupe seeds. It is similar in nutrient and benefit profile to **watermelon seed oil**. It is very light and easily absorbed, making it useful for all skin types. Able to be used undiluted or in combination with other oils, it is generally used in face creams, face oils, and face serums targeting acne and aging.

Mustard oil (genera *Brassica* and *Sinapis*): This oil is extracted from mustard seeds. Although there is controversy about using it internally, and it is actually banned for internal use in some countries, it is considered safe for topical use. It is rich in **essential fatty acids**, **vitamin C**, and **antioxidants** and has antibacterial, antifungal, and antiviral properties. Beneficial for extremely dry, cracked, and brittle hands, feet, and nails, it also reduces fine lines and wrinkles, removes dark spots, alleviates cold symptoms, promotes hair growth, and helps protect against UV damage. Not considered suitable for undiluted use, it is often added to massage oils, hair oils, face masks, face oils, bath soaks, and salves.

Mustard seeds (genera *Brassica* and *Sinapis*): Soft and round yellow mustard seeds are used whole as a gentle **exfoliant**. They're also added to salt scrubs for additional exfoliation as well as primarily used in hard bar soaps for gentle spherical exfoliation that also gives the soap an added boost of cleansing power.

Myristic acid: This saturated fatty acid is used as a **surfactant** and **emulsifier**, and in perfumes. It can be derived from both animal and vegetable sources and is found in many products such as face masks, cleansers, soaps, and lotions.

Myrrh essential oil (*Commiphora myrrha*): Extracted from myrrh resin, this very expensive essential oil is used for both perfume and essential oil blends, generally in small quantities due to its price. Traditionally it is used medicinally for its anti-inflammatory, antibacterial, antiviral, and sedative properties. It is found in skin care targeting acne or signs of aging.

Myrrh hydrosol (*Commiphora myrrha*): This hydrosol has all the benefits of myrrh essential oil and the extract in a less caustic form. It can be used undiluted and to replace water in formulations to impart both the scent and efficacy without the cost. It is very soothing for skin and often used as a toner.

Myrrh resin extract (*Commiphora myrrha*): Extracted either in an oil or solvent, this is a less expensive and less concentrated alternative to myrrh essential oil.

N-acetyl L-tyrosine: This substance is primarily used as an **antioxidant** and conditioner to protect and replenish skin. It can be found in cosmetic products such as serums, moisturizers, and conditioners. It's also used as a tanning agent, though there is little data on this ingredient.

Nanoparticles: These are microscopic particles with at least one dimension of less than 100nm. The cosmetic industry has been embracing nanotechnology for its ability to deliver a more profound application. For example, in natural sunscreens zinc oxide is often used. With normal zinc oxide particulates, the sunscreen will be opaque and greasy, but when nanoparticles are used it is less oily, has a better texture, and penetrates the skin more deeply. However, nanoparticle use is controversial because the extremely small size means they get absorbed into body and skin tissue and can cause cell destruction and potentially even environmental pollution. Little is known about the safety of using nanoparticles.

Narcissus absolute: Narcissus absolute is made by a solvent extraction and is a very rare and expensive absolute. It is generally used in small amounts in antiaging face care products for its exotic scent and ability to repair.

Narcissus poeticus bulb extract: This extract contains a wide range of compounds that boost the immune system and are antiviral, anti-inflammatory, and anticancer. In skin care, the extract is used in antiaging products to decrease inflammation and reduce premature aging. It also has a positive effect in the treatment of acne.

Narcissus poeticus wax: This wax is used as an **emollient** and thickening agent, and to add a smooth and creamy texture. It is used in body lotions and face creams to repair, restore, and protect skin from environmental damage. It also has a calming and relaxing effect.

Neem oil: The oil is cold-pressed from the fruit and seeds of the tropical neem tree. It is high in **essential fatty acids** and **antioxidants** and has anti-inflammatory, antifungal, antiviral, and antibacterial properties. It is also a pesticide. It visibly reduces redness and inflammation and has been used in traditional medicine as a remedy for acne and viruses because of an aspirin-like compound that combats bacteria. It can be mildly irritating for some skin types and should never be used undiluted. While its effects are profound for skin, its strong aroma makes it challenging to formulate within a significant percentage.

Neopentyl glycol dicaprylate/dicaprate: This is a synthetic combination of neopentyl glycol and a blend of fatty acids. The fatty acid components help lubricate skin and increase cell resilience. It's used as an **emollient** and texturizer in products such as concealers, lipsticks, conditioners, foundations, and cleansers and has been classified as safe for cosmetic use.

Neroli essential oil (*Aurantium amara*): This extremely expensive essential oil comes from the blossoms of the bitter orange tree native to tropical regions in Asia and Africa. It should never be applied undiluted but added to a product in a small percentage or used with a carrier oil. The scent is highly desirable, but due to cost, it is generally used in a very small percentage in a larger scent blend.

Neroli extract (*Aurantium amara*): Due to the scarcity and expense of both **neroli essential oil** and **hydrosol**, this extract, which carries little to no scent, is often used in skin care for its **antioxidant**, anti-inflammatory, and soothing properties as a way of achieving some of the benefits without the cost. It is added to products containing the oil or hydrosol to boost benefits and decrease the amount of oil or hydrosol needed.

Neroli hydrosol (*Aurantium amara*): Neroli hydrosol is an **antioxidant**-rich, purifying astringent that has soothing properties that can regenerate skin cells, decrease redness, maintain elasticity, and rejuvenate skin. It also fights inflammation and is antibacterial, making it helpful in the treatment of both acne and rosacea. It is

gentle and can be used undiluted on all skin types. Alone, it makes a wonderful toner or facial mist. It can also replace water in any formulation to increase efficacy.

Niaouli essential oil (*Melaleuca quinquenervia*): This tree is related to the tea tree. Niaouli is considered a milder version and is suitable for sensitive skin. Its antiseptic properties are beneficial in the treatment of oily and acne-prone skin. It is also used for detoxifying and uplifting mood.

Noni (*Morinda citrifolia*): This evergreen tree in the coffee family was originally grown in the tropics. Clinical studies have shown that noni guards against and decreases wrinkles; visibly reduces crow's-feet; and improves skin health, elasticity, tone, and firmness to maintain a youthful glow.

Nonoxynols: These are used for **surfactants**, solvents, and **emulsifying** agents. There is potential contamination with known carcinogen ethylene oxide and formaldehyde donor 1,4 dioxane. While deemed safe for rinse-off products, they are a controversial ingredient. They can be found in almost every type of cosmetic from body lotions and hair care to face creams and bubble bath.

Nutmeg essential oil (*Myristica fragrans*): Studies have shown nutmeg to be antibacterial, antiviral, and **antioxidant**, although the most studied attribute is its calming effect on the nervous system. It is used for its aromatherapeutic properties as well as in hand sanitizers and for acne. Some people can have a sensitivity to the essential oil, so it's important to patch test it before use.

Nutmeg powder (*Myristica fragrans*): This powder is used in face masks and exfoliators targeting acne. Generally, people with acne should not exfoliate with manual **exfoliants**. Cut and sifted powder is used in facial steams targeting breakouts and blackheads.

Nutmeg wax (*Myristica fragrans*): This exotic wax has a different profile from most waxes and adds a warm, spicy note to products. It is calming and used in bar lotions, lip balms, and face and body care. It is also used in body creams and salves for pain relief. It provides skin conditioning, viscosity, firmness, and stability.

Nylon-12: A synthetic polymer that is both solid and flexible, this is a popular bulking agent and texture and viscosity enhancer. It is used in many products from cosmetics and fragrances to soaps and face and body creams.

O-cymen-5-ol: A synthetic preservative used in cosmetics, this controversial ingredient has been deemed safe for use in cosmetics in America in a 0.5% concentration, although Europe has approved it for only 0.1%. Additionally, some studies done in the 1950s found it neurotoxic to animals. Currently, information is limited.

Oak bark (*Quercus cortex*): Oak bark contains tannins and is a gentle astringent. It also has anti-inflammatory and antibacterial properties that have a positive effect on dermatitis and inflammation of the skin. It is used in bath soaks and salves aimed at reducing inflammation, and is added to facial toners.

Oak moss essential oil (*Evernia prunastri*): This is a species of lichen. Oak moss fragrance is often called an essential oil, however it is not made by steam distillation but by chemical solvent extraction.

The essential oil is generally used in fragrances and scent blends. It is a controversial ingredient, and the EWG rates it 7/10 for toxicity.

Oak moss extract (*Evernia prunastri*): The extract has **antioxidant**, antibacterial, antiviral, and antifungal properties. It is extracted with light heat process in either **glycerin** or oil. It does not have the same aroma as the essential oil and is generally used in hand sanitizers, shampoos, skin care targeting acne, as a fragrance ingredient, and in foot care. Natural skin care companies wanting the benefits of oak moss will often opt for the oil or glycerin extraction instead of the "essential oil," despite its different aroma.

Oat extract (*Avena sativa*): A member of the grass family, oats can be used as a natural cleanser that visibly soothes, calms, and softens. Studies have shown that colloidal oatmeal provides a protective barrier against irritants and holds moisture in. It also acts as an **emollient**, balances pH, and reduces itchiness. Oats have **antioxidant** and anti-inflammatory benefits and protect against UV radiation. Oat extract is used in skin care, bath and body care, and is often combined with colloidal oatmeal.

Oat oil (*Avena sativa*): Derived from entire oat kernels by a solvent extraction, this nongreasy oil has **antioxidant** and anti-inflammatory properties. It is easily absorbed by skin and used in acne treatments.

Oat straw extract (*Avena sativa*): This benefits of oat straw are less well known than the edible oat, but it has potent effects on skin. The extract is made from the dried stalks, leaves, and tops of oat plants and used for its nutrient content of vital minerals such as calcium, magnesium, and silica. Oat straw tincture is used in skin care and hair care to provide a restorative mineral boost. It helps regulate skin's oil production and is anti-inflammatory, so it soothes and calms red, itchy, irritated skin. It is used in skin care aimed at excessively oily skin and sensitive skin.

Obsidian clay (illite): Obsidian clay is a purifying clay rich in natural minerals including sulfur, which makes this clay beneficial for skin conditions such as acne, eczema, or psoriasis. Its high absorption capacity makes it very helpful for oily skin and for deep-cleaning pores. It purifies skin and visibly reduces the appearance of blemishes and breakouts.

Octinoxate: A common ingredient used for its ability to absorb and filter UV rays, octi-noxate is used in face creams with SPF, sunscreens, and to preserve the freshness of other ingredients. There are safety concerns as research has shown reproductive and developmental issues for expectant mothers; it is also a penetration enhancer. It is often found in products targeting acne, although some researchers found it can cause breakouts and dermatitis. The FDA states there is not enough evidence to consider it harmful to humans and has not restricted it in cosmetic use, although consumers and natural skin care companies consider it controversial.

Octyl palmitate: Derived from palm oil, this ester is used for viscosity and to add a thick and creamy texture. It is also used as a silicone replacement as it gives skin the same silky, polished feeling. It can clog pores and increase breakouts.

Octyldodecyl myristate: This compound is used as a thickening agent and **emollient**. There is little information on its safety, and currently it is deemed nontoxic.

Oenocarpus bataua fruit oil: Extracted from the fruit of a palm tree native to the Amazon rain forest, this oil's extensive fatty acid profile contains antibacterial, **antioxidant**, and antiviral properties, along with amino acids, **essential fatty acids**, and **vitamin A**. It is used in skin care for moisturizing, to combat acne, and as a thickening agent and an antiaging ingredient. It is easily absorbed by skin, leaving a nongreasy feel.

Oenocarpus bataua extract: This extract is made from a combination of the bataua fruit leaves and roots, which both contain **antioxidants** although the leaves contain more. It is used in skin care to prevent damage from UV rays and environmental stress, reduce signs of aging, and prevent fine lines and wrinkles.

Olive leaf extract (Olea europaea): Tradi-tionally, this oil pressed from the fruit has been used in skin care. Less common but highly effective, the leaf extract is gaining popularity for its antibacterial, anti-inflammatory, **antioxidant**, and antiviral properties. One potent antioxidant present in large amounts, oleuropein, makes the extract highly effective in protecting against free radical damage, collagen deterioration, and aging. The extract is used topically to treat acne and wrinkles, as well as a preservation booster.

Olive oil (Olea europaea): Olive oil is rich in one of the few natural sources of the super hydrating and **emollient** squalene. The oil has an abundance of **essential fatty acids** and **antioxidants**. It also stops overproduction of oil and is used for eczema, psoriasis, and postoperative scar tissue. As well as maintaining a proper moisture balance, it aids in elasticity and healing severely chapped and cracked skin. Olive oil is noncomedogenic and penetrates deep into the skin to provide profound, long-lasting moisture and help skin stay smooth, soft, and supple. Olive oil is used in body lotions, face creams, face oils, and soap. It can be used in cold-process soaps. The more olive oil, the less lather, so it is generally combined with other oils.

Olive pomace oil (*Olea europaea*): Olive pomace oil is a by-product of olive oil production. It has some of the same nutrient profile but is much less concentrated and not as beneficial for skin. It is less expensive than regular olive oil and primarily used for soapmaking. As with regular **olive oil**, this can be used in cold-process soaps, though usually in combination with other oils.

Orange extract (*Citrus × sinensis*): Oranges contain more than 170 phytochemicals and are packed with **antioxidants**. The extract is generally made from the peel, which has the highest concentration of antioxidants. It protects skin from UV damage and helps revitalize collagen and support skin structure. Orange extract is a noncaustic way to get the benefits of the orange peel without the scent of the essential oil.

Orange juice (*Citrus sinensis*): Orange juice is high in **antioxidants** and helps maintain youthful skin, reduce wrinkles, prevent collagen deterioration, and eliminate dead skin cells. It can replace water in skin care formulations or be added to hard bar soaps.

Orange peel (*Citrus sinensis*): Orange peel contains powerful **antioxidants** that protect skin from environmental stressors, purify and rebalance skin, and visibly reduce signs of aging. It has antiseptic properties and encourages growth of new skin cells, so it is commonly used to treat stretch marks and other forms of damaged skin. Dried and powdered peel is also used in face masks.

Oregano essential oil (*Origanum vulgare*): Extracted from oregano leaves, this essential oil contains carvacrol, which is antibacterial; thymol, an antifungal; and rosmarinic acid, an **antioxidant**. These three ingredients make a powerful combination to treat acne, athlete's foot, and topical infections, although its strong odor makes it difficult to use in concentrations high enough for full efficacy.

Oregano extract (*Origanum vulgare*): Made from oregano leaves (sometimes with the seeds), the leaf extract can be in alcohol or chemical solvents. It contains all the benefits of the essential oil in a less concentrated and pungent form.

Oregano hydrosol (*Origanum vulgare*): Oregano hydrosol is antiseptic, antifungal, and antiviral. It has all the benefits of the essential oil in a less caustic form and can be used undiluted or to replace water in a formulation to increase efficacy. The aroma is less strong than the essential oil but still strong enough that it generally is blended with something else. It is often used in foot soaps and acne products as well as hand sanitizers, deodorants, and sometimes mouthwash.

Oregano seed oil (*Origanum vulgare*): Filled with **essential fatty acids**, **antioxidants**, and **vitamin E**, this oil also contains antifungal and antibiotic properties. It is used in antiaging products to hydrate skin and help it retain moisture, visibly reduce signs of aging, protect skin against environmental damage, and maintain healthy collagen.

Orris root: This ingredient is generally from the roots of *Iris germanica* and *Iris pallida*. It is used for its beautiful violet-like aroma as a fixative in perfumes, essential oil blends, and in powders, potpourri, bath salts, and facial steams.

Oryzanol: This is an ester used for its skin-conditioning, softening, and anti-aging benefits in face creams, masks, face oils, and serums for mature skin.

Oxidoreductase: An enzyme that increases the efficacy of **antioxidants** used in products to prevent signs of aging, oxidoreductase facilitates the anti-oxidants in preventing the breakdown of collagen and elastin and protecting against environmental damage. It is anti-inflammatory and can be used on sensitive skin.

Ozokerite wax: A naturally occurring paraffin found in shales and sandstones, this is a fairly hard wax with **emulsifying** and **emollient** properties that is often used for viscosity and thickness in many products.

Palm kernel oil (*Elaeis guineensis*): This comes from the same plant as palm oil but is extracted from the seed rather than the flesh. Filled with **antioxidants**, it is used in antiaging creams and soaps.

Palm oil (*Elaeis guineensis*): From the flesh of the fruit of the oil palm, palm oil is dark orange due to the high levels of car-otenes. It contains **essential fatty acids** and tocotrienols, strong **antioxidants** that help fight free radicals, visibly reduce fine lines and wrinkles, and cleanse without a greasy feel. It is primarily used in soapmaking, body lotions, and products for antiaging.

Palmarosa essential oil (*Cymbopogon martini*): Extracted from the leaves of a plant native to southeast Asia, this essential oil has antibacterial and antiviral properties and is used for acne, balancing oil produc-tion, eczema, dry and oily skin, psoriasis, wound healing, wrinkles, and infections.

Palmarosa hydrosol (*Cymbopogon martini*): This hydrosol has all the beneficial properties and scent of palmarosa essen-tial oil but in a less caustic form that can be used undiluted or to replace water in formulations to increase efficacy. It is very versatile and beneficial for all skin types, making it popular in a wide variety of face care products. It is effective for eczema and psoriasis and used in sprays and bath soaks targeting the treatment of both.

Papaya (*Carica papaya*): Native to Mexico and South America, papaya contains an enzyme called papain, which removes dead skin cells to resurface skin. Papaya is a rich source of **antioxidants** that protect skin from environmental factors, wrinkles, and aging.

Papaya seed oil (*Carica papaya*): Extracted from papaya seeds, the oil contains **essential fatty acids**, **antioxidants**, and enzymes. It is also antibacterial and antifungal and is used to treat acne and athlete's foot. It is added to face cleansers to help remove dead skin cells and rejuvenate skin, face oils to protect against aging and acne, and to scalp oils and foot balms.

Parabens: Parabens are a group of synthetic chemicals used as preservatives in cosmetics and personal care products. They include butylparaben, propylpara-ben, methylparaben, isobutylparaben, and ethylparaben. Despite much press about their toxicity, the FDA considers them safe for use. Some studies argue that cumulative exposure contributes to health problems, including risk of breast cancer as they're said to disrupt hormone function.

Parsley seed essential oil (*Petroselinum crispum*): This essential oil has the benefits of parsley seed oil in a more concentrated form. It should be diluted before use. It is generally used in wound care and is becoming a popular ingredient in products targeting acne.

Parsley seed oil (*Petroselinum crispum*): Extracted by cold-pressing, this very pure oil is gaining popularity. In comparison to other oils it has one of the strongest capacities to protect against free radical damage. It is filled with phytochemicals and **essential fatty acids** and is used in skin care to fight and reverse signs of aging, and to treat acne.

Passion fruit oil (*Passiflora edulis*): Passion fruit oil comes from the seeds of the passionflower plant, native to South America and Africa. It is full of vitamins and nutrients including **vitamins A** and **C**, copper, magnesium, calcium, **carotenoid**s, and **essential fatty acids**. It is an extremely hydrating, lightweight, nongreasy, and noncomedogenic oil, making it suitable for all skin types. It protects skin against environmental damage and premature signs of aging, reduces the appearance of fine lines and wrinkles, and keeps skin smooth and supple.

Patchouli essential oil (*Pogostemon cablin*): Extracted from the leaves and stems of a plant in the mint family, this essential oil has an earthy, woody scent that is used in perfumes and essential oil blends for face care and body products. Topically, it has astringent, antifungal, antibacterial, and wound-healing properties and is used for acne, eczema, dermatitis, and dandruff.

Patchouli hydrosol (*Pogostemon cablin*): Patchouli hydrosol has all the attributes of the essential oil in a less caustic form and can be used undiluted. The scent is similar to the essential oil but a bit more fresh and vibrant. It is used in toners and cleansers for acne, shampoos, deodorants, and body sprays for eczema and psoriasis.

Pawpaw fruit (*Asimina triloba*): Pawpaw fruit, from a small deciduous tree native to Canada and the United States, is antibacterial and high in **antioxidants**, magnesium, and amino acids. It gently removes skin cells and helps protect collagen and maintain healthy skin. The fruit is used in skin care products for antiaging and acne.

Pawpaw seed oil (*Asimina triloba*): This oil, extracted from pawpaw seeds, is high in **essential fatty acids** and found in many products from face oils and creams to soaps. It is used to treat dehydrated skin, eczema, and psoriasis.

Peach flesh/juice (*Persica vulgaris*): Peaches are anti-inflammatory and contain **antioxidants** such as quercetin, **vitamin C**, and potassium. They are used topically to reduce wrinkles, smooth skin texture, maintain and promote new healthy collagen, protect against environmental damage, and help remove dead skin cells. They can be used either fresh or powdered in face masks, facial cleansers, face creams, and soap.

Peach kernel oil (*Persica vulgaris*): This oil is extracted from the peach kernel. It has a shorter shelf life and is less stable than other oils. It is high in **essential fatty**

acids and amino acids and is used in facial products for antiaging.

Peanut oil: Extracted through cold-pressing, peanut oil is pure and retains the beneficial nutrients, although refined oil (bleached and deodorized) is often used as it is generally considered safe for those with peanut allergy. It is filled with **essential fatty acids**, **vitamin E**, and amino acids. It is intensely hydrating, protects skin from UV radiation, and helps maintain the skin's natural protective barrier.

Pear seed oil (*Pyrus communis*): Pear seed oil is harvested from pears, whereas **prickly pear oil** is harvested from cacti. This oil, which is lightweight and quickly absorbed, visibly improves skin elasticity and restores moisture to leave skin feeling smooth and soft. It is used in face creams and oils as a powerful ingredient for antiaging.

Pecan meal (*Carya illinoinensis*): Pecan meal has all the properties of the oil plus the ability to exfoliate without causing microdermabrasions. It is used in face **exfoliants** in cream or powdered form, which avoids the need for preservatives in formulations. It is also used in soapmaking to provide gentle exfoliation.

Pecan oil (*Carya illinoinensis*): Cold-pressed from the nuts and rich in **essential fatty acids** and **vitamin E,** pecan oil is nongreasy and easily absorbed by skin, where it protects against UV damage, hydrates, and helps generate new skin cells. It is used in face care products targeting dehydration, mature skin, and visible signs of aging.

Pectin: This gelatinous **polysaccharide** that naturally occurs in fruits is used as a thickener, gelling agent, and texture enhancer. Often, apple pectin is used in skin care as it also has the benefits of the **antioxidants**, **alpha hydroxy acids**, and other attributes of apples.

PEG: This is an acronym for polyethylene glycol. There are many PEG compounds as polyethylene glycol can be mixed with fatty alcohols or fatty acids to create different ingredients. Each has a different use in cosmetics, such as being **emollients** or **surfactants**. Depending on the manufacturing process, ingredients formulated with PEGs may be contaminated with carcinogenic ethylene oxide and formaldehyde-donor 1,4 Dioxane. 1,4 Dioxane can be removed during manufacturing but, as with all PEGs, there's no way to know whether the PEGs has undergone that additional process. PEGs are also penetration enhancers, allowing all ingredients in a product more profound transdermal access.

PEG-7 glyceryl cocoate: This ester is made from **glycerin** and **coconut oil**. It is used as a thickening agent, foam booster, **emollient**, and for skin conditioning. Product labels may be confusing and state "all natural derived from glycerin and coconut oil" when in fact it contains manufactured **PEG**.

PEG 8: This is the ester of **lauric acid** used as both a **surfactant** and **emulsifier**. (*See PEG for safety concerns.*)

PEG 14: This is a polymer of ethylene oxide. PEG 14 is used as a skin-conditioning agent. It can clog pores and cause irritation. (*See PEG for safety concerns.*)

PEG 32: This **emulsifier** is used to suspend oil and water. (*See PEG for safety concerns.*)

PEG 33: This is used as a **humectant** and solvent and for viscosity. (*See PEG for safety concerns.*)

PEG 90M: Used to add lubrication and viscosity and for film forming, this also helps stabilize **emulsions**. (*See **PEG** for safety concerns.*)

PEG-100 stearate: Also known as polywax, this is used as an **emulsifier**. It is made by combining oils with stearic acid (a naturally occurring fatty acid in plants and animals) or ethylene oxide and fatty acids. Ethylene oxide is a carcinogen and traces of the by-product 1,4 dioxane (a formaldehyde donor) can remain in the product. The substance is used in creams, lotions, and conditioners. (*See **PEG** for safety concerns.*)

PEG-150 distearate: A polyethylene glycol diester of stearic acid (a naturally occurring fatty acid in plants and animals). It is both a thickener and **surfactant** and used in products such as shampoo, bubble bath, and shower gel. It can also be used with other **emulsifiers** in lotions and creams. (*See **PEG** for safety concerns.*)

Peppermint extract (*Mentha* x *piperita*): This extract is primarily used in skin care products such as facial cleansers to control oil production, and as an anti-inflammatory and mild astringent.

Peptides: Peptides are a chain of amino acids linked by amide bonds (peptide bonds). While there is exciting research about their benefits, some of it has been exaggerated, such as marketing it as a replacement for cosmetic surgery. Although they are often used alone, peptides work best in skin care formulations when in conjunction with other ingredients such as **antioxidants**.

Perilla seed oil (*Perilla frutescens*): This oil comes from the seeds of a plant in the mint family native to Asia. It is rich in **essential fatty acids**, including omega-3.

It has antibacterial and anti-inflammatory benefits as well as being a potent **antioxidant**. It is readily absorbed into the skin, nongreasy, and noncomedogenic, making it particularly useful for treating acne, aging, and dehydrated skin.

Petitgrain (*Citrus aurantium* var. *amara*): Often called poor man's **neroli**, petitgrain is derived from the same tree as neroli but extracted from the leaves and twigs rather than the blossom. It is much less expensive than neroli and therefore more widely used in perfume and essential oil blends. Topically, it effectively treats acne and bacterial infections and can be used as an antiseptic, to balance oil production, and heal wounds. It is safe for sensitive skin.

Petitgrain hydrosol (*Citrus aurantium* var. *amara*): The hydrosol is widely used as it has all the aroma and attributes of the essential oil but can be used undiluted or to replace water in formulations to increase efficacy and impart scent. It is suitable for sensitive skin. It calms redness and inflammation and eases rosacea. It is used in toners, face cleansers, face creams, and body lotions and also as a calming and relaxing spray.

Petrolatum/petroleum: Petroleum can be found on many skin care product labels under such names as xylene, toluene, mineral oil, and liquid paraffin. Besides being comedogenic, there are safety concerns as it contains 1,4 dioxane, a probable carcinogen.

PHA (polyhydroxy acids): AHA (**alpha hydroxy acid**) and BHA (**beta hydroxy acid**) are commonly found in many skin care products. PHAs are less well known but considered a better choice for sensitive skin as their molecular structure is larger so they don't penetrate skin as easily. They are **humectants** and they gently exfoliate and dissolve dead skin cells.

Phenoxyethanol: This lesser-known preservation alternative to **parabens** became popular when parabens started getting negative press. However, there is evidence of its harmful effects, and many natural skin care companies now choose to be phenoxyethanol free as well as paraben free.

Phenylalanine: Occurring naturally in high-protein foods such as eggs, meat, and milk, phenylalanine has amino acids and lipids and is used for skin conditioning, hydrating, and to visibly reduce signs of aging. There's some conflicting information about taking it internally as a supplement, and although it is generally considered safe, people with PKU (phenylketonuria) need to avoid it.

Phenylpropanol: Phenylpropanol is used for preservation against bacteria, yeasts, and molds. It can cause skin sensitivity and in a study, rats dosed orally with 3-phenylpropanol at certain levels died within two days. While considered safe by many natural skin care companies, there's insufficient research on its safety. It is used in products that are both left on and rinsed off, such as lotions or cleansers.

Phthalate: Phthalates are generally used to make plastics, but they're also used as solvents. The long-term health effects are not conclusive, but research has shown them to affect the reproductive system in laboratory animals; more research is being done to confirm the findings and ascertain safe levels of use and exposure. Currently the FDA does not require a listing of the individual ingredients of fragrance, so phthalates may end up in products but not be labeled. They're

generally found in nail polish, fragrances, and hair care products.

Phytic acid: Phytic acid naturally occurs in plant seeds. Its use internally is controversial as it impairs the absorption of minerals. Seeds can be soaked, sprouted, or fermented to reduce the phytic acid content. Topically, it is used as a powerful **antioxidant** in skin care products aimed at reducing signs of aging.

Phytonutrients: Plants contain different chemicals called phytonutrients. This large group of chemicals helps the plant survive by protecting it from fungus, bugs, and other elements. There are more than 25,000 phytonutrients that are powerhouse ingredients for skin care, doing everything from decreasing dehydration and wrinkles to protecting against environmental stressors and retarding signs of aging.

Pine bark extract (*Pinus sylvestris*): Pine bark has anti-inflammatory, antibacterial, and antiviral properties. The extract can either be extracted in an oil or a chemical solvent and used as an antiaging agent and to treat acne.

Pine essential oil (*Pinus sylvestris*): Made from pine needles, this essential oil is antiseptic and detoxifying and used for eczema, psoriasis, cuts, sores, congested pores, and acne. It is often found in facial toners, body creams, bar lotions, and salves.

Pine leaf extract (*Pinus sylvestris*): Extracted either in oil or a chemical solvent, pine leaf extract has been studied for efficacy against cancer cells. There is less research about its effect on skin. It has **antioxidant** properties and is found in some toners, cleansers, and face creams.

However, some people have a sensitivity to it.

Pineapple (*Ananas comosus*): Pineapple contains bromelain, an enzyme that softens skin, visibly reduces the appearance of inflammation, removes dead skin cells, and combats buildup. Perfect for problem skin, the enzyme helps disintegrate excess surface cells for efficient and nonabrasive exfoliation, leaving skin clean and luminous. It also helps hydrate skin and improves elasticity.

Pink kaolin clay: This is a mixture of white and red kaolin clays. It offers all the properties of both clays, although it does not have the absorption capacity of the red alone. Its beautiful color and attributes make it popular for face and body masks. Clays are often used in soaps and this pink clay gives soap a lovely natural color.

Pink lotus absolute (*Nelumbo nucifera*): The flower from which this oil comes is also known as the sacred lotus or water lily. It is used for hyperpigmentation, muscle pain, antiaging, and as an astringent. This popular ingredient is included in perfumes and scent blends in everything from body lotions and massage oils to soaps and face creams.

Pink lotus leaf extract (*Nelumbo nucifera*): Made from pink lotus leaves, this extract is filled with **bioflavonoids** and **antioxidants**. It protects skin against environmental damage, slows signs of aging, helps reduce fine lines and wrinkles, and prevents sagging. The powdered form is advantageous for face masks and **exfoliants** in the natural skin care sector as it eliminates the need for preservation systems; the liquid form is used in face creams and body lotions.

Pistachio nuts (*Pistacia vera* L.): Pistachios contain **essential fatty acids**, amino acids (in higher concentration than most other nuts), vitamins, minerals, **antioxidants**, and **phytonutrients**. They're also prebiotic. The nuts are ground into a flour and used as a gentle **exfoliant**, in powdered face masks, and soapmaking. They're beneficial for all skin types, including sensitive.

Pistachio oil (*Pistacia vera* L.): This oil has the same nutrient profile as the nuts in a more concentrated form. It's light, nongreasy, noncomedogenic, and easily absorbed into skin. It is beneficial for all skin types and used in everything from lotions and body creams to face oils and soaps.

Plankton extract: Plankton extract comes from a combination of marine skeletons, seaweeds, and algae. Rich in vitamins, amino acids, minerals, and silica, it is used for its soothing, intensively moisturizing, antiaging, antiwrinkle, and anticellulite abilities. It also helps maintain healthy collagen structure and promotes renewal.

Plantain fruit (*Plantago major*): Originally native to Europe and Asia, plantains are extremely high in **vitamin C** and potassium and are useful for a range of skin types. They lock in moisture and soothe dry, flaky skin while promoting healthy cell development, resulting in a glowing complexion. By stimulating the natural rejuvenation process, they can also diminish acne scars, balance skin tone, and act as a natural protectant for healing skin.

Plantain leaf (*Plantago major*): Plantain leaves are soothing **emollients** packed with powerful anti-inflammatories that make them valuable for topical wound healing and for acne, and antiaging products.

Plum kernel oil (*Prunus domestica*): Extracted from plum kernels in a cold-press process without using solvents, this pure oil is high in **essential fatty acids** and **antioxidants**. It can be used undiluted but generally is combined with other oils. It is most effective when used for dehydrated skin as well as an antiaging agent.

Plum vinegar: The popularity of apple cider vinegar in skin care has paved the way for other vinegars, such as this one, which is also known as umeboshi vinegar. Plum vinegar is rich in **antioxidants** and enzymes that digest skin cells, help balance pH, and protect against aging. It is used in facial toners, cleansers, and masks.

Polyethylene: This synthetic wax made from ethylene is a type of plastic used in products for stability, hardness, and as a thickening agent. It is used in stick formulations such as lipstick, foundation sticks, and sunscreen sticks; it enables these products to withstand heat. It also helps prevent oil separation and creates a film to make colors more vibrant.

Polyhydroxystearic acid: This very soft wax derived from the castor plant (see **castor oil**) is used as a thickening agent, to increase viscosity, hardness, and to form a film. It adds a creamy texture and stability to **emulsions**. It's used in color cosmetics, sunscreens, gels, and body creams.

Polypodium leucotomos: This potent **antioxidant** comes from a fern that grows in Central America. It inhibits the growth of free radicals and prevents damage from UV radiation. It's a powerful anti-inflammatory and helps in the production of new skin cells and the repair of damaged skin cells. It is used to treat psoriasis and prematurely aging skin.

Polysaccharides: These are carbohydrate molecules composed of a variety of sugar molecules bonded together. They give lotions and creams better spreadability and a decadent feel. They increase hydration levels, decrease fine lines and wrinkles, and even out skin tone. They may also have **antioxidant** properties.

Polysorbate 20: This is one of the most common **emulsifiers** used as an **emollient**, **surfactant**, and stabilizer in cleansers, moisturizers, and skin care products for children. The carcinogen ethylene oxide, and traces of 1,4 dioxane (a formaldehyde donor) can remain in the product.

Polysorbate-60: This is an **emulsifier** consisting of sorbitol (a sugar alcohol), ethylene oxide (a carcinogen), and stearic acid (a naturally occurring fatty acid in plants and animals). Research shows it is a mild skin and eye irritant. It is typically considered to be a low hazard ingredient; however, there are concerns regarding cancer risks and reproductive toxicity (the EWG group rates it 3/10).

Polysorbate-80: This is an **emulsifier** consisting of sorbitol (a sugar alcohol), ethylene oxide (a carcinogen), and oleic acid (a fatty acid). It has the ability to penetrate the blood-brain barrier and potentially cause anaphylactic shock. It also caused reproductive abnormality in rats. Some consider this controversial ingredient safe; others suggest it should be avoided.

Pomegranate juice (*Punica granatum*): This juice is packed with minerals and vitamins, especially **vitamin C**, and contains **antioxidant** and anti-inflammatory properties that protect and defend skin and hair against harmful elements such as UV rays, stress, poor diet, and pollution that damage and prematurely age skin and deteriorate collagen.

Pomegranate peel extract (*Punica granatum*): Pomegranate peel is made into an extract and used in high-end skin care. It has a stable shelf life, unlike the juice and oil, but more importantly it has a more concentrated ratio of **antioxidants** and anti-inflammatories, providing the benefits of the seed and the oil in higher concentration. It lacks the **essential fatty acids** present in the oil and is often combined with creams and oils to increase the benefits.

Pomegranate seed oil (*Punica granatum*): Pomegranate seed oil contains **essential fatty acids**, **antioxidants**, and anti-inflammatories and is often paired with **pomegranate peel extract** as it increases the delivery of the active ingredients. Research has shown it to be effective on skin tumors.

Poppy seed oil (*Oleum papaveris seminis*): Used both internally and topically, this oil is rich in **vitamin E**, **antioxidants**, and **essential fatty acids**. It is fairly stable with a longer shelf life than most plant oils and is used in face oils and creams targeting aging and dehydration.

Poria cocos extract: Also known as *hoelen* and *fu ling*, this extract is from an edible mushroom traditionally used medicinally. It contains anti-inflammatory, **antioxidant**, antibacterial, and antiviral properties, plus amino acids. Its ability to regulate oil production makes it effective for oily and acne-prone skin. It is also used for mature, sensitive, or dehydrated skin, and to visibly reduce signs of aging.

Potassium phosphate: This inorganic salt is used to adjust pH and as a buffering agent.

Potassium sorbate: Used as both a food grade and a cosmetic preservative, this substance derived from petroleum is suspected of causing allergies in some people and has been found to have negative health effects. It offers no skin-enhancing qualities. Previously popular as a natural preservation system, more companies are looking for an alternative. The EWG now gives it a 3/10 on its hazard rating.

Pracaxi seed oil (*Pentaclethra macroloba*): From an evergreen tree native to tropical areas in South America, this oil is extremely high in **essential fatty acids**, is anti-inflammatory and antibacterial, and helps generate new skin cells. Due to its nutritional profile it is suitable for many applications but is generally used in skin care products targeting dehydration and acne.

Prickly pear oil (*Opuntia ficus-indica* L.): Extracted from the seeds of a member of the cactus family, prickly pear oil is rich in **vitamins A** and **C**, calcium, and potassium, as well as tannins, **flavonoids**, and alkaloids. It increases cell renewal.

Probiotics: Probiotics are microorganisms that contribute to and promote health and balance in their host. They are found in foods such as yogurt, kefir, sauerkraut, and kombucha. While many forms are not vegetarian or vegan, there are vegan sources of probiotics. Probiotics help protect skin against external contaminants, balance pH, are anti-inflammatory, help reduce acne breakouts, and retard signs of aging. They have also been shown to prevent free radical damage, which accelerates skin aging and collagen deterioration. For skin health they are used both internally as well as topically in skin preparations such as face creams and serums.

Propanediol: This is used to control the viscosity of a product, for conditioning, and as a **humectant** and preservation booster. One of the biggest concerns is its manufacture and the potential environmental and health effects. One method of manufacture is from acrolein, which is also found in cigarette smoke and may be a factor in lung cancer. Often cited as "natural," propanediol can be made from genetically modified (GMO) corn. The most widely used version in the cosmetic industry comes from DuPont Chemical. It's found in products from masks and shampoos to moisturizers and sunscreen.

Propolis: This sticky substance is made by bees from sap, beeswax, and other elements they use as a coating to build their nests. It contains **antioxidants** specifically high in **flavonoids** and is also considered to be antibacterial, antifungal, anti-inflammatory, and antiviral. It is used in salves for wound healing and scars, in acne products, and in antiaging skin care.

Propylene glycol: This petroleum-derived substance is a penetration enhancer. It's a suspected immune system, reproductive, skin, and respiratory toxin. It is extremely common and found in hair care products, lotions, shower gels, and deodorants. There is no efficacy or benefit from using this for skin.

Pumice powder: Pumice stones are naturally produced from volcanic ash. The stones are milled to a very fine powder and used in foot scrubs, hand scrubs, and soaps to remove excessive dirt and oils, and dead skin (especially on feet). It may be found in facial scrubs but is considered too abrasive and should be avoided.

Pumpkin flesh (*Cucurbita pepo* L.): All parts of the pumpkin are used in skin care for their different attributes. The flesh is rich in **beta-carotene** and also contains enzymes, **alpha hydroxy acid**, vitamins, and minerals. It is also a power booster for other ingredients. The molecular structure of pumpkin is small, giving it exceptional transdermal penetration and allowing it to carry other ingredients in a product with it. The flesh can be dried and powdered and used in face masks, body scrubs, and facial **exfoliants**.

Pumpkin seed (*Cucurbita pepo* L.): Rich in natural enzymes and **alpha hydroxy acids**, pumpkin seed helps remove dead skin cells, giving skin a smoother and brighter appearance. They also contain **essential fatty acids** that replenish lost moisture. Pumpkin seeds are finely ground and used as a very gentle **exfoliant** or added to cleansers. They are suitable for all skin types.

Pumpkin seed oil (*Cucurbita pepo* L.): Cold-pressed from the seeds, pumpkin oil is packed with **vitamin E**, zinc, **antioxidants**, and omega-3 and -6 fatty acids to boost collagen and protect against signs of aging. **Essential fatty acids** hydrate skin while regulating oil production and fighting acne. Studies have shown the oil to be beneficial in healing wounds and burns. It helps maintain a healthy skin barrier, which protects skin from environmental stressors and damage. It is beneficial for all skin types, including sensitive.

Pumpkin stem cells (*Cucurbita pepo* L.): Plant stem cells are currently hot ingredients in skin care, and while some studies cite the benefits of pumpkin stem cells, most agree that more research is needed.

Companies, however, are increasingly adding plant stem cells to products as consumers are seeing the results.

PVM/MA decadiene crosspolymer: This synthetic polymer is used as a binding agent and thickener.

PVP (polyvinylpyrrolidone): This synthetic water-soluble polymer is used in cosmetics for stabilizing, viscosity, binding, and film forming.

R

Raspberry flesh (*Rubus idaeus* L.): Raspberries are currently considered a superfood due to their high levels of **antioxidants** and anti-inflammatories. For skin care, the whole berries are dried and ground, which enables the beautiful pink color to be imparted to products such as soaps, face creams, bath soaks, face masks, and bath bombs.

Raspberry juice (*Rubus idaeus* L.): Raspberry juice contains the nutrients of the berry in a concentrated form. Being liquid, it has more versatility than the powder and can be used in everything from creams and soaps to shampoo and face serums. It also contains a higher level of natural fruit sugars (**AHAs**), which remove dead skin cells and rejuvenate skin.

Raspberry seed oil (*Rubus idaeus* L.): Extracted from the seeds, this oil is rich in **antioxidants**, **essential fatty acids**, and nutrients that repair, hydrate, soften, smooth, protect, and condition skin. It is noncomedogenic, nongreasy, and easily absorbed. It is a highly versatile oil that can be used on all skin types, including sensitive, from head to toe.

Red algae (*Ahnfeltia concinna*): This easily absorbed algae imparts nutrients to skin, hydrating, moisturizing, revitalizing, and maintaining skin health, elasticity, structure, and youth.

Red clover (*Trifolium pratense*): Red clover has been used medicinally internally for respiratory problems associated with colds and flu and for symptoms of menopause. It is also now being used in salves, bath soaks, and aromatherapy blends for these symptoms. Topically, it calms inflamed skin. Rich in vitamins and minerals, it is most commonly used in skin care to treat psoriasis, eczema, and rashes.

Red currant (*Ribes rubrum*): These small red fruits are filled with macronutrients such as protein, fats, natural fruit sugars, **vitamins C** and K, iron, and **antioxidants**. They help maintain collagen structure, slowing signs of aging, preventing sagging, and helping generate new skin cells. They also protect skin against environmental damage.

Reishi mushroom extract (*Ganoderma lucidum*): This extract can be found in organic alcohols and is filled with bioactive compounds and **antioxidants** that protect skin against contaminants, generate new skin cells, maintain healthy collagen structure, and slow signs of aging.

Reishi mushroom powder (*Ganoderma lucidum*): This powder is gaining popularity due to its efficacy and ability to be formulated in face masks and facial **exfoliants** without the use of water, which negates the need for a preservation system. Containing only dried ground mushroom, it is more concentrated than the extract. The powder is used in soapmaking and provides gentle exfoliation as well as skin softening and soothing.

Reishi mushroom spore oil (*Ganoderma lucidum*): This oil extracted from the mushroom spores has the highest concentration of **triterpenes**, which heal and repair skin. It is used for acne, dehydrated skin, wound healing, scar reduction, and mature skin.

Reishi mushroom water (*Ganoderma lucidum*): Mushroom water can replace water in formulations to increase efficacy and impart the benefits. Reishi mushroom water is not only a powerful antiaging ingredient for mature skin but is also an **emollient** that leaves skin incredibly soft and supple.

Resveratrol: This compound is found in large concentration in red wine, grape skins, blueberries, cranberries, and peanuts. It is popular in skin care for its **antioxidant**, anti-inflammatory, and antiaging properties and is used in face creams and serums targeting premature aging, wrinkles, and fine lines.

Retinaldehyde: This gentler form of **vitamin A** requires only a single-step conversion to retinoic acid, the active form cells can use, which may lead to faster visible results. Though not conclusive, studies suggest that, like **retinol**, retinaldehyde can aid in cellular turnover yet cause very little, if any, irritation. Because it's more widely tolerated, it can be beneficial for those with sensitive skin wishing to take advantage of vitamin A's antiaging and acne-fighting properties.

Retinoids: This generic term covers a class of potent chemical compounds derived from synthetic **vitamin A**. Brand names for this prescription-only ingredient include Retin-A and Differin. Studies show that when applied topically (usually in a cream) retinoids are accepted directly into skin cells. This makes them extremely effective in diminishing the appearance of fine lines, wrinkles, hyperpigmentation, and stretch marks, while also fighting acne. That said, they can be highly irritating, causing redness, peeling, and photosensitivity. Pregnant women or women who may become pregnant are advised against using retinoids.

Retinol: Retinol is the alcohol form of synthetic **vitamin A** that's available over the counter. Less effective than **retinoids**, retinol is still a powerful ingredient that accelerates cell renewal. It can be seen in antiaging and acne-targeted skin care formulations such as moisturizers and serums. It's known to cause irritation in some people and should not be used by pregnant women.

Retinyl palmitate: This synthetic ester of **retinol** and palmitic acid is a less potent **vitamin A** derivative that requires high concentrations for efficacy. It can be found in a variety of products, including lipsticks, sunscreens, foundations, moisturizers, serums, shampoos, and conditioners. Many products that contain it may not have enough in their formulations to achieve any visible results. That said, pregnant women are still advised against using it.

Reverse osmosis water: Since water can comprise up to 80% of a formulation, skin care companies look for pure options to maintain quality and efficacy. It also is helpful when labeled so people can identify the source of the water when assessing the quality of the product. While reverse-osmosis water is a pure form of water and beneficial for skin care, most eco-friendly companies choose not to use it as it takes about 4 gallons of water to produce 1 gallon.

Rhassoul clay: Mined from Morocco, this ancient clay has a high mineral content. It's effective at drawing out impurities, old oils, dirt, and debris and improving skin texture and elasticity. It is suitable for all skin types.

Ribwort plantain (*Plantago lanceolata* L.): Ribwort, a flowering perennial in the plantain family, contains tannins that provide gentle astringency, polysaccharides, and anti-inflammatories that provide emollient and soothing, calming benefits. Studies have shown that it has significant anti-inflammatory properties when used topically.

Rice bran oil (*Oryza sativa oleum*): Extracted from the germ and interior of the rice husk, this easily absorbed, very light oil is rich in **essential fatty acids**, squalene (**emollient**), and **antioxidants**. It is used in antiaging face creams and oils.

Rice flour (*Oryza sativa oleum*): Rice flour naturally softens and gently removes dead skin cells from the face and body. It is often used in spa treatments and soapmaking.

Rice starch (*Oryza sativa oleum*): An inexpensive common ingredient and alternative to cornstarch, rice starch is used as a filler in face masks, for viscosity in lotions, and in makeup and body powders. Like cornstarch, when applied and left on the skin its natural sugars encourage the growth of yeast and can activate acne, diaper rash, and redness.

Rice syrup (*Oryza sativa oleum*): Generally made from whole-grain brown rice that's treated with enzymes, then boiled into a syrup with a honey-like consistency, rice syrup has amino acids, **essential fatty acids**, natural sugars, vitamins, and minerals. It is used as a facial cleanser and **exfoliant**, and in face masks.

Rice water (*Oryza sativa oleum*): Made by soaking and sometimes gently simmering rice, rice water is used in face creams to treat psoriasis and eczema and to promote soft, supple, and velvety skin. It is also used in face cleansers and to dissolve and remove dead skin cells.

R-lipoic acid: This is the natural form of lipoic acid (**AHA**). It is not as commonly used in skin care but some consider it to be superior. This **antioxidant** is highly touted for its ability to penetrate both oil and fluid, thus giving it greater transdermal penetration and higher efficacy.

Rock rose absolute (*Cistus ladanifer*): This absolute is derived through a solvent extraction that makes it less expensive than the essential oil. Since it still retains all the attributes it can replace the essential oil.

Rock rose essential oil (*Cistus ladanifer*): This essential oil is used for mature skin, acne-prone skin, congested skin, and eczema. Studies have shown it to be effective as a wrinkle reducer, as an antibacterial, and for eliminating pore buildup.

Rock rose extract (*Cistus ladanifer*): This extract has antifungal properties and is rich in tannins. It does not carry the scent of the essential oil or the absolute and is used in cleansers and toners targeting acne as well as in salves and creams for feet.

Rock rose twig hydrosol (*Cistus ladanifer*): Made from the twigs of the rock rose plant, this hydrosol can be used undiluted or to replace water in formulations to increase efficacy. It is most often used for mature skin for its firming and toning effects as well as its ability to repair and reduce signs of aging. It is very gentle and calms irritated, red skin, rosacea, and acne.

Roman chamomile essential oil (*Anthemis nobilis* L.): From a perennial plant native to Europe and Africa, this essential oil is used to treat headaches, acne, wrinkles, insomnia, muscle pain, anxiety, eczema, psoriasis, cold sores, and joint pain. Generally, it is used in a very low percentage in face oils and creams for acne or antiaging, body lotions and bath soaks for psoriasis, eczema, and in salves for pain.

Roman chamomile extract (*Anthemis nobilis* L.): This extract is used for its anti-inflammatory, **antioxidant**, antiaging and pain-management properties to help treat acne, wrinkles, eczema, redness, irritation, and rashes. It helps calm and sooth sensitive skin.

Roman chamomile hydrosol (*Anthemis nobilis* L.): This hydrosol carries the same properties as the essential oil in a non-caustic form that can be used undiluted or to replace water in formulations to increase efficacy. It is often included in face creams to combat acne, dehydration, and wrinkles, or as a toner or facial mist.

Rooibos: This is a **flavonoid** and **antioxidant** superstar that is gaining momentum in the skin care industry. Intensely purifying and pore decongesting, the extract and tea are used in acne products and creams for dehydration and eczema for their antibacterial and anti-inflammatory properties. It is suitable for all skin types, even extremely sensitive.

Rosa canina hip extract: Generally extracted in alcohol, this extract contains **flavonoids**, tannins, fatty acids, **carotenoids**,

vitamin C, amino acids, calcium, and **alpha hydroxy acid**. It's important to know exactly what it is extracted in to ensure it contains no toxic components. It is used in antiaging skin care, to help protect skin against UV damage, and to replenish skin cells and collagen.

***Rosa canina* hip oil:** Also known as rose hip, this oil is naturally rich in **antioxidants**, intensely hydrating, and quickly absorbed. Rose hip contains retinoic acid (**vitamin A**), which helps promote protein synthesis and cell regeneration. Increasing skin's capacity to produce new tissue can diminish the appearance of fine lines and wrinkles.

***Rosa canina* hydrosol:** This 100% pure plant product is used for its ability to reduce signs of aging and improve tone and firmness. Naturally scented, its joyful scent lifts spirits while working wonders on skin.

***Rosa canina* leaf extract:** *Rosa canina* leaves contain alkaloids and **saponins**. The leaf extract is generally used in cleansers and toners targeting the effects of aging.

***Rosa canina* leaf oil:** This oil is made by a hydro-distillation process that results in a product more similar to an essential oil than a hydrosol; it has a similar profile to **rose leaf extract**.

***Rosa canina* seed powder:** Rosa canina seeds are milled or ground to a very fine powder that will gently remove dead skin cells. It is gentle enough to use alone or in facial cleansers and masks aimed at resurfacing skin.

***Rosa x centifolia* extract:** Also known as cabbage rose, this extract is used for its **antioxidant**, anti-inflammatory, and astringent properties. It helps condition skin, decongest pores, and protect skin from free radical damage.

Rosa x centifolia flower wax: Obtained from the flowers of a cabbage rose hybrid, this wax carries a lovely faint rose scent that it imparts to products. It is generally used in high-end antiaging skin care.

Rosa x damascena absolute: This absolute is produced by a solvent, making it less expensive and more readily available, although it is generally used for the same applications as the essential oil.

Rosa x damascena essential oil: Extracted from a great many roses, the very small amount of essential oil produced is used to calm nerves, calm and repair skin, and relieve PMS symptoms and depression.

Rosa x damascena extract: This is the extract of a concentrated form of both the hip and the flower. Knowing what it was extracted in is important when selecting products. The extract is a very versatile and inexpensive form of the rose, making it widely used in many face care and body care products.

Rosa x damascena flower wax: Derived from the flower petals, this wax has the beautiful rose aroma. It is used as an **emollient** and for creaminess and texture in products such as lip balms, face creams, and body lotions.

Rosa x damascena flowers: The dried flowers, which contain **antioxidants** and anti-inflammatories, are either used whole as buds or petals, or powdered. The buds or petals are used in facial steams, bath teas, or added to products for their decorative quality. The ground powder is used in face masks and **exfoliants**.

Rosa x damascena hips extract: Rich in vitamins, minerals, **essential fatty acids**, and tannins, this extract has a potent profile without the scent of the essential oil or the absolute. It is used for its ability to protect skin from free radical damage, repair and treat collagen, and reduce signs of aging. The hips can also be ground and powdered or cut and sifted. The powder is used in face masks and facial **exfoliants**, and the cut and sift is used in facial steams and bath teas.

Rosa x damascena hydrosol: This hydrosol, with its fairly strong and vibrant aroma, has become one of the most popular rose waters. It helps calm sensitive skin, reduces redness, protects skin from damage, and is used as a facial toner or in lotions and creams to increase efficacy.

Rose geranium essential oil (Pelargonium roseum): Used for its aroma in perfumes and products such as body lotions and face creams, this essential oil is antimicrobial and antifungal and beneficial in acne products, foot salves, hand sanitizers, and deodorants.

Rose geranium extract (Pelargonium roseum): Made from the stem and leaves of this flower, extract is used for pain and depression and as an antibacterial, antifungal, and **antioxidant**.

Rose geranium hydrosol (Pelargonium roseum): This hydrosol has all the attributes of the essential oil in a less concentrated form and can replace water in formulations to increase efficacy. It is used for acne toners and cleansers as well as foot soaks and lotions.

Rosemary essential oil (*Rosmarinus officinalis*): Filled with **antioxidants** and anti-inflammatories, this herbaceously scented essential oil decreases muscular pain. It is often added to lotions, soaps, and creams where its primary use is for oily, acne-prone, and aging skin.

Rosemary extract (*Rosmarinus officinalis*): Made from rosemary needles and filled with **antioxidant**, antimicrobial, and anti-inflammatory properties, this extract does not have the potency or aroma of the essential oil, which widens its applications and makes it a useful, nonfragrant addition to face creams and oils targeting the effects of aging, oily skin, and acne.

Rosemary hydrosol (*Rosmarinus officinalis*): This hydrosol contains the same benefits as the essential oil but in a noncaustic form that can replace water in formulations to increase efficacy. It is filled with nutrients that protect skin from UV and free radical damage; reduce breakouts, pore size, and excessive oil; and visibly tighten skin. It can be used undiluted as a facial toner or body mist.

Rosewood essential oil (*Aniba rosaeodora*): Made from rosewood, this essential oil is antibacterial, antiseptic, and naturally stimulating. Its scent is added to perfumes and essential oil blends. Topically, it is used to decongest pores, for acne, oily skin, inflammation, psoriasis, scars, and cell regeneration.

Rosewood extract (*Aniba rosaeodora*): This antifungal, antibacterial, and antiviral extract is generally extracted in alcohol and used in deodorants, hand sanitizers, and acne products.

Rosewood hydrosol (*Aniba rosaeodora*): This hydrosol has all the benefits of the essential oil in a less caustic form and can be used undiluted. The pure hydrosol is used as a base for natural deodorant, in acne toners, as a tension headache–reducing spray, for psoriasis, and to help control oil production.

Royal jelly: Secreted by bees and fed to the queen and larvae, royal jelly contains abundant nutrients including vitamins, minerals, **antioxidants**, antibacterials, and anti-inflammatories. It supports and hastens wound healing, increases healthy collagen production, and slows signs of aging. It's used internally as a supplement as well as being a staple in skin care.

Sacha inchi oil (*Plukenetia volubilis* L.): From a perennial vine native to the Peruvian rain forest, this new and increasingly popular oil contains a super high concentration of **essential fatty acids** including omega-3 and omega-6, **vitamins A** and **D**, and other nutrients. It is noncomedogenic, and helps decongest pores, and its **antioxidant** properties are highly effective for antiaging.

Saccharide isomerate: This carbohydrate is used for its ability to increase hydration, moisturize, and keep skin soft and supple.

***Saccharomyces* lysate:** This is a yeast compound used as a conditioning agent and **antioxidant** to increase moisture levels in skin. Although yeast and yeast-derivative ingredients are becoming very popular in skin care, there is little documentation on their efficacy.

Safflower seed oil (*Carthamus tinctorius*): An annual plant grown commercially for the oil extracted from the seeds, this oil can be cold-pressed or refined. The finished oil is packed with **essential fatty acids** and **antioxidants** that visibly increase skin's elasticity and reduce the appearance of wrinkles. It protects skin against environmental damage and premature aging. It is noncomedogenic, easily absorbed, inexpensive, and readily available. An effective moisturizer, it can substitute for widely used oils such as almond oil in nut-free applications.

Saffron (*Crocus sativus*): Derived from a resilient flower that can thrive in extreme conditions, saffron protects skin against environmental damage. Studies have shown that using saffron at 4% concentration garners 8% SPF. It is also a soothing **antioxidant** and anti-inflammatory.

Sage (*Salvia officinalis* L.): Native to the Mediterranean, sage has a very strong aroma and is often used for its aromatherapeutic attributes. Used topically, it is an astringent, antibacterial, anti-inflammatory, and antifungal and is typically used in toners, deodorants, and foot soaks.

Sage hydrosol (*Salvia officinalis* L.): Sage hydrosol is gently astringent and has antibacterial and anti-inflammatory attributes that make it beneficial in the treatment of acne. It can replace water in any formulation to boost the product's active profile and can be used undiluted as a facial toner.

Sake: This traditional Japanese alcoholic beverage is made by fermenting rice. It has natural sugars and enzymes that help gently exfoliate. It is also used for brightening skin, which is different from lightening skin, in that it restores glow. It can be added to bathwater or replace a proportion of water in skin care products to boost efficacy. It's generally used in face cleansers, toners, or masks.

Sal seed butter (*Shorea robusta*): Extracted from the seeds of an evergreen tree that grows in India, sal seed butter is a true butter with no added ingredients. It is filled with **essential fatty acids**, amino acids, minerals, and vitamins. Because it is hard butter, it can be used in smaller percentages to add thickness and viscosity to a body cream or lotion. It is also used in foot creams, salves, lotions, and lip balms.

Sal seed flour (*Shorea robusta*): Made from the seeds by defatting the kernel to make powder, sal seed flour is filled with amino acids, tannins, and minerals and used as a gentle **exfoliant** in facial cleansers, face masks, and soaps.

Saponins: These are a group of carbohydrates that naturally occur in certain plants such as yucca, ginseng, licorice, and soap nuts. They are natural **surfactants** and **emulsifiers** and soothe skin; most contain **antioxidants**.

Savory (*Satureja bachtiarica*): Antibacterial, antiviral, **antioxidant**, and anti-inflammatory, savory contains **flavonoids** and is generally used in cleansers, toners, and face serums targeting acne.

Savory essential oil (*Satureja bachtiarica*): This essential oil is antiseptic, analgesic, antibacterial, and filled with **antioxidants**. Its herbaceous aroma is used in perfume and essential oil blends. Topically it is used to treat acne and in hand sanitizers and deodorants.

Saw palmetto extract (*Serenoa repens*): Extracted in either alcohol, **glycerin**, oil, or chemical solvents from the berries, this extract is available in both powder and liquid form and is used in face masks, cleansers, and toners targeting acne.

Saw palmetto oil (*Serenoa repens*): This oil is extracted from the berries but is cold-pressed and therefore very pure and rich in **essential fatty acids**. It is used in products targeting acne and, unlike the extract, can be used in face oils.

Schisandra berry extract (*Schisandra chinensis*): Research being done on this extract's benefits for antiaging has had promising results. The extract appears in products aimed at balancing moods, and it is also beginning to be found in face creams targeting wrinkles and other signs of aging.

Sea buckthorn berries (*Hippophae rhamnoides*): All parts of this deciduous plant are used medicinally for different purposes. The berries are used to ward off infections and retard aging and to prevent sunburn, dry skin, and eczema. They are used in skin care for dehydrated, acne-prone, and prematurely aging skin.

Sea buckthorn leaves and flowers (*Hippophae rhamnoides*): The leaves and flowers of this plant are often combined and used for treating joint pain, rashes, and acne. They are a valuable source of many vitamins, **antioxidants**, proteins, fatty acids, and minerals and are used in salves to target inflammation and pain, and in products to generate collagen and combat acne and aging.

Sea buckthorn oil (*Hippophae rhamnoides*): This intensely concentrated oil contains all the benefits of the berry. It is **antioxidant**, anti-inflammatory, and a rich source of **vitamins C, A, E, and beta-carotene** as well as minerals, amino acids, and fatty acids. It is noncomedogenic, highly **emollient**, easily absorbed, and used to repair collagen, protect from environmental damage, reverse and retard signs of aging, and combat dehydrated skin.

Sea salt: Sea salt is produced through the evaporation of ocean water or water from saltwater lakes, usually with little processing. Depending on the water source, the evaporation leaves behind certain trace minerals and elements. Sea salt rejuvenates skin and improves blood circulation while moisturizing, detoxifying, and revitalizing.

Seaweed: There are many types and varieties of seaweed used in skin care. Overall they commonly provide hydration, visibly reduce inflammation and signs of aging, and help remove toxins. They also fight against free radical damage, protect collagen from deterioration, and repair and mend. They're often added as an extract, which is a more concentrated form than seaweed itself.

***Senna alata* leaf extract:** From a shrub grown throughout Thailand, these leaves are used for their antifungal properties; studies have shown them to be effective in the treatment of skin issues with fungal activity. Topically, the extract is used to treat dandruff, acne, and psoriasis.

Sesame seed (*Sesamum indicum*): Originally grown in tropical regions and traditionally used as a culinary condiment, sesame seeds have made their way into skin care products. They are an excellent source of calcium, magnesium, iron, zinc, selenium, amino acids, **antioxidants**, and **essential fatty acids**. The seeds are very high in oil and therefore hard to make into powder, but the ground seeds are used as an **exfoliant** in soaps, facial scrubs, and cleansers.

Sesame seed oil (*Sesamum indicum*):
This oil has the concentrated nutrient profile of the seeds. It is easily absorbed by skin, noncomedogenic, and intensely moisturizing. It is anti-inflammatory and used in massage oils to alleviate pain. It also protects skin against UV radiation and environmental damage, making it an important oil in antiaging products. Both toasted and untoasted sesame oils are available for culinary purposes, but for skin care formulations, cold-processed untoasted oil is used.

***Sesbania grandiflora* bark:** This bark is an astringent and used in facial toners and facial cleansers.

***Sesbania grandiflora* leaves:** These leaves contain amino acids, **antioxidants**, **flavonoids**, antibacterials, anti-inflammatories, and antivirals. They are used in an array of products: in bath soaks and salves to reduce inflammation and heal bruises and in acne and antiaging skin care.

Shea butter (*Butyrospermum parkii*): This oil (butter) is extracted from the nuts of a tree native to Africa. It is generally refined, bleached, and deodorized for skin care preparations. Rich in fatty acids and **vitamins A, E**, and F that visibly reduce inflammation, nourish, and moisturize, it is also filled with powerful **antioxidants** and anti-inflammatories that rejuvenate, oxygenate, and offer a protective barrier. An effective moisturizer, it can be used undiluted on hands, elbows, lips, and feet to prevent and heal cracking and severe dryness, as well as added to body lotions and soaps.

Shea oil (*Butyrospermum parkii*): This rare oil comes from the same source as **shea butter** and is very similar to the butter except for being liquid, which gives it different applications. Like the butter,

it has an extremely high **essential fatty acid** content and is used for moisturizing, in hair care, and for dehydrated skin. Its liquid form means it is often used in massage oils, bath oils, and body lotions.

Shiitake mushroom (*Lentinula edodes*): These edible mushrooms contain vitamins, minerals, amino acids, **polysaccharides**, and **antioxidants**. As well as being used medicinally in supplements, topically they are anti-inflammatory and antiaging and are becoming a mainstay in skin care. The mushroom is dried and powdered and used in face masks and facial **exfoliants**.

Shiitake mushroom extract (*Lentinula edodes*): This extract is much more powerful than the plain mushroom and can be used in a greater variety of products. It is a powerful antiaging ingredient and helps prevent dehydration, wrinkles, crows'-feet, sagging, and discoloration.

Shiitake mushroom water (*Lentinula edodes*): Derived from soaked and sometimes partially heated mushrooms, this water softens and soothes skin as well as removes dead skin cells, increases cellular turnover, protects collagen, and reduces signs of aging. It can replace water in face and body creams or serums, and is used in soapmaking. When making mushroom soap, the soaked mushrooms are pulverized and added to the soap along with the water.

Silica: Silica is one of the most abundant elements found on Earth and in the human body. Topically, silica helps produce new collagen and skin cells, which improves elasticity, tone, and strength.

Silica microbeads: An alternative to plastic microbeads, this biodegradable product can be added to skin care products for gentle exfoliation.

Silk amino acids (*Bombyx mori*): Silkworms produce a protein, sericin, that research shows has significant effect on wound healing as well as imparts **antioxidants**. Its ability to repair and mend tissue means it is beneficial in products geared toward treating acne. It is also used for antiaging products with the combined benefits of antioxidants and protein. It protects skin against environmental damage and promotes collagen renewal.

Skullcap (*Scutellaria baicalensis*): This purple flowering perennial plant contains a powerful **antioxidant** and anti-inflammatory profile that includes intense free radical scavengers. It also offers skin-brightening properties and is a popular ingredient in skin care products for acne, eczema, psoriasis, and antiaging.

Slippery elm bark extract (*Ulmus rubra*): Traditionally, the bark of this tree native to the United States and Canada has been used medicinally. It is a natural **mucilage**, and when used in skin care it softens, soothes, and conditions.

Smithsonite extract: This extract is from the semiprecious stone, which is rich in zinc sulfite and is being touted for its antiaging ingredients that have an effect similar to Botox. While gemstones may be all the rage in skin care, there's little substantiating scientific data to confirm their effectiveness.

Sodium benzoate: Sodium benzoate is widely used in natural skin care cosmetics as part of a preservation system and also used as a food-grade preservative. Several studies have linked it to health issues. While not a harmful ingredient alone, when combined with ascorbic acid it creates a chemical reaction that forms benzene, a chemical used in pesticides, hair dyes, plastics, and that is also in secondhand smoke. The American Cancer Society deems it a known carcinogen, so it should be avoided.

Sodium bicarbonate: This salt raises the pH of bathwater. Research suggests that a pH level closer to ocean water (8) could be beneficial to skin and help remove dead skin cells, though as an **exfoliant** sodium bicarbonate is too rough and should not be used in facial scrubs. It is an antibacterial. While it is often used in acne treatments it is beneficial only for spot treatment, without scrubbing. It is used in fizzing bath products, bath soaks, and body scrubs.

Sodium coceth sulfate: This **surfactant** is used as a milder alternative to **sodium laureth sulfate**. It is derived from the fatty acids of **coconut oil** and modified using ethylene oxide (a carcinogen); traces of 1,4 dioxane (a formaldehyde donor) can remain in the product. It is used in products that lather and often used in baby products.

Sodium hydroxide: This inorganic compound is also known as lye and is used for making cold-processed soap. A lye-and-water bath is mixed with fats for the saponification process to create soap. Pure lye is caustic and precautions need to be taken, but finished soap does not contain any lye as it is converted to a new compound during the soapmaking process.

Sodium laureth sulfate: Made from either petroleum or **coconut oil** and potentially contaminated with 1,4-dioxane (a formaldehyde donor) this is the most widely used detergent and **surfactant**. Negative press about this ingredient means companies are looking for better alternatives.

Sodium PCA: Derived from amino acids, this **humectant** is naturally found in human skin. Research shows it has the ability to bind moisture in the air to hair and skin cells to maintain hydration. Found in products such as shampoos, conditioners, cleansers, and moisturizers, it is considered safe for cosmetic use in concentrations up to 4%.

Solar-evaporated Pacific sea salt: Harvested off the Pacific Coast and solar evaporated, these pure small granules of salt cleanse, balance oil production, and combat bacteria. Traditionally used in body scrubs and bath salts, it is also showing up in deodorants and acne sprays.

Sorghum bicolor: Sorghum is a tall grass native to Africa. It is used as a natural colorant for soap. It is filled with vitamins and has **antioxidant** and anti-inflammatory benefits.

***Sorghum bicolor* stalk juice:** Sorghum bicolor stalk juice is antibacterial, antiviral, and **antioxidant** and contains vitamins and minerals. It gently removes dead skin cells and gives a boost to dull, lackluster skin.

Soy milk: Filled with amino acids, **essential fatty acids, isoflavonoids,** vitamins, and minerals, soy milk can be used in skin care either powdered or fresh. It maintains collagen structure and health, generates new cells, removes dead skin cells, and softens and soothes skin. It is used in many products from face creams and body lotions to bath salts and bath bombs.

Spearmint essential oil (*Mentha spicata*): Extracted from spearmint leaves, this essential oil contains menthol, anti-inflammatories, antifungals, **antioxidants, bioflavonoids,** and other vitamins and nutrients. It is highly concentrated and can irritate skin and eyes, so it is generally used in very small amounts in lotions, soaps, massage oils, and body scrubs. Its cooling effect makes it useful in pain-relieving salves and lotions.

Spearmint hydrosol (*Mentha spicata*): Spearmint hydrosol has all the benefits of the essential oil but is nonirritating. It is often used in acne toners and cleansers as well as antiaging cleansers, as it helps stimulate skin. Because it is nonirritating, the hydrosol can be effectively used in the treatment of psoriasis.

Spirulina (*Arthrospira platensis*): This blue-green algae found in oceans throughout the world is commonly used internally as a supplement. It is anti-inflammatory, antiviral, and is packed with protein, vitamin B12, **vitamin A**, iron, and **essential fatty acids**. Since it lacks cell walls, its nutrients are easily accessed by skin. It increases skin hydration and leaves a breathable protective barrier. It also helps balance oil production. It is a widely used ingredient in skin care products of all kinds.

Squalane: Naturally produced in sebum, squalane lubricates skin, but body levels begin to decline rapidly from our early twenties. It is a highly effective **emollient** and a powerful **antioxidant** that prevents damage from UV rays, increases cellular turnover, promotes collagen strength, prevents age spots, and is antibacterial, nongreasy, easily absorbed, and good for all skin types. It can be obtained from oils such as olive and amaranth.

St. John's wort extract (*Hypericum perforatum* L.): The plant is grown worldwide for medicinal properties, for its oil, and also for its flowers. Topically, this extract is used for its antibacterial, anti-inflammatory, and **antioxidant** properties. Due to its mood-enhancing properties it is added to bath soaks aimed at calming and relieving stress. The extract is also used in small quantities in face creams and serums.

St. John's wort oil (*Hypericum perforatum L.*): This oil is extracted from the flowers, which impart a beautiful red color, and is generally very expensive. It is used to calm sensitive, red, irritated skin, making it a wonderful addition to acne products. It is also used to treat eczema and severely dry skin.

Stinging nettle (*Urtica dioica*): These leaves, flowers, and roots are used in extracts for skin and hair. It is **antioxidant**, anti-inflammatory, and mineral rich, making it beneficial in products geared toward antiaging. It protects against cellular and UV damage, slowing wrinkles and fine lines. It has also been shown to be effective in wound healing.

Strawberry (*Fragaria ananassa*): Strawberries are grown worldwide for their fruit, which contain **flavonoids**, **vitamin C**, folic acid, and potassium. The fresh pulp and juice as well as powdered strawberries are used in skin care products. Strawberries are anti-inflammatory and slightly astringent; they help loosen dead skin cells, protect skin from environmental damage, and brighten skin. They're primarily used in antiaging products such as face creams, face masks, and cleansers.

Strawberry seed oil (*Fragaria ananassa*): Made by a cold process that does not include refinement, this very pure oil has antibacterial and **antioxidant** properties and an intense ability to condition, moisturize, and help skin stay hydrated.

It is very soothing, making it suitable for all types of skin, including sensitive. It is readily absorbed and can be used undiluted but is generally combined with other oils. Most beneficial for acne-prone and aging skin, it is used in face creams, oils, and massage oils.

Sugandha bala essential oil (*Pavonia odorata*): Extracted from the rhizomes of a perennial herb native to India, Pakistan, Burma, Sri Lanka, and Africa, the essential oil has antibacterial, antiviral, and antifungal properties. It is used in skin care targeting acne as well as in massage oils, deodorants, hand sanitizers, and foot creams.

Sugandha bala extract (*Pavonia odorata*): The extract is anti-inflammatory, antiviral, and antibacterial. It is mainly used for its anti-inflammatory benefits in bath soaks and pain-relieving cream as well as in antiaging face care.

Sugar, raw (*Saccharum officinarum*): Although considered much healthier than processed sugar, raw sugar is processed in the same manner until the final stages. This leaves a gentle coating of molasses on the raw sugar. It has the same attributes for skin care as white cane sugar with an additional mineral boost from the molasses.

Sugar, white cane (*Saccharum officinarum*): The **AHAs** in white sugar rejuvenate and resurface skin, remove dead skin cells, and help maintain moisture. High levels of AHAs can be irritating and cause redness and sensitivity in some types of skin. Sugar granules are used for body and face **exfoliants**. They are square and have sharp edges, but when they're mixed with water and applied to skin the edges soften, preventing microdermabrasions or tears. Sugar exfoliants should be avoided on acne-prone skin.

Sugar, white cane juice (*Saccharum officinarum*): Extracted from the sugarcane plant, the juice is a concentrated, less-processed form of sugar granules. Being liquid, it can be added to different products such as cleansers, face masks, creams, and serums. It is often used as a gentle option to impart **AHAs**.

Sulfates: These comprise a large group of ingredients used in products primarily for their ability to lather and bubble. They are detergents that can irritate skin.

Sunflower seed oil (*Helianthus annuus*): Extracted by either cold or heat methods, the oil is squeezed from the hulled seeds. Warm-pressed seeds result in better yields. Sunflower seed oil contains **essential fatty acids** and linoleic acid and improves cell regeneration. It also moisturizes, and is noncomedogenic and anti-inflammatory.

Sunflower seed wax (*Helianthus annuus*): The sunflower seed wax is obtained from the winterization of sunflower seed oil. Winterization means removing the higher melting point parts, such as waxes. It is used as a natural thickening agent, for viscosity, and to give stability, smoothness, solidity, and a creamy texture to products such as lipsticks, creams, lip balms, bar lotions, and color cosmetics.

Sunscreen chemicals: Some chemicals such as oxybenzone, homosalate, octinoxate (octylmethoxycinnamate), octisalate, and octocrylene cause hormone disruption, skin allergies, and other issues. Some have transdermal penetration and have been found in mothers' milk. The two with the most negative research results are oxybenzone and octinoxate.

Surfactant: These controversial ingredients are lathering and foaming agents. They're used to break down oils and fats, enabling them to be cleansed from skin. Getting luscious lather naturally is difficult. Often, labels stating natural surfactants will add "derived from coconut/sugar or . . ." which sounds good, but neither coconut nor sugar lather when added to water. The result of the original derivative is far from either coconut or sugar.

***Syzygium cumini* bark extract:** With its fatty acid, **flavonoid**, and tannin content, the extract is used in facial toners and cleansers as a gentle and mild astringent that helps remove oils and debris and is suitable for sensitive skin.

***Syzygium cumini* essential oil:** The essential oil contains **essential fatty acids** and **antioxidants**. Anti-inflammatory and antibacterial, it is used in products treating acne and signs of aging, and in balms targeting psoriasis and eczema.

***Syzygium cumini* flower:** Also known as Java plum, this plant is in the myrtle family and native to the tropics. Its flowers are rich in **flavonoids** and **antioxidants**. It is an extremely soothing and calming ingredient used to help reduce redness and in the treatment of psoriasis, eczema, and rosacea.

***Syzygium cumini* fruit:** The fruit is not only a natural source of **antioxidants**, it also contains **anthocyanins**, **flavonoids**, amino acids, calcium, natural fruit sugar, mineral salts, and **vitamin C**. The extract from the fruit is used in facial cleansers, face masks, and antiaging and hydrating face creams.

Syzygium cumini **leaves:** Rich in **bioflavo-noids** and **antioxidants,** the leaves are used in products targeting aging and to protect against free radical damage.

Syzygium cumini **root:** The root is rich in **flavonoids** and often mixed with other parts of the plant to increase potency in antiaging skin care products.

Tabernaemontana divaricata **L.:** Also known as pinwheel flower or crepe jasmine, this evergreen shrub native to India has been shown to have antibacterial, antiviral, and **antioxidant** properties. It is being added to skin care products targeting aging and acne.

Table salt: Typically mined from underground salt deposits, table salt is heavily pro-cessed to eliminate minerals and usually contains an additive to prevent clumping. Most table salt also has added iodine. Traditionally, table salt is not used in skin care although it is less expensive than sea salt, so some companies use it as an alternative in bath soaks and body scrubs.

Talcum powder: A naturally occurring min-eral, talcum powder has long been used as baby powder and as an absorbent in makeup such as eye shadow, blushes, and foundation. Talc itself is not a harmful substance, but it is often contaminated with asbestos, a known carcinogen.

Tamanu oil (*Calophyllum inophyllum***):** Produced from the seed of the tropical tamanu tree, the oil has extremely high fatty acid content and **antioxidant,** antifungal, anti-inflammatory, antibacterial, and antiviral properties. It easily penetrates all layers of skin, helps

skin regenerate, and visibly reduces blemishes and scarring. For face care, it is generally recommended to dilute it.

Tamarillo (*Cyphomandra betaceae***):** The edible fruit is filled with powerful **antioxidants** and **flavonoids** and is used to protect collagen, protect skin against environmental stressors, reduce the appearance of wrinkles, and exfoliate dead skin cells. It is most often found in extract form and added to face creams and serums, although powder made from the fruit and seeds is used as an **exfoliant.**

Tarragon essential oil (*Artemisia dracunculus***):** Tarragon is a perennial herb in the sunflower family. Although anti-inflammatory and antiviral, the essential oil is not often used in skin care as it can cause sensitivity and contains some phytochemicals that may be carcinogenic. It is not recommended for DIYers.

Tartaric acid: This **alpha hydroxy acid** can be made synthetically or from grapes. The synthetic form is the most commonly used form in skin care. It is an effective **exfoliant** and may be tolerated more easily than **glycolic, lactic,** and **malic acids,** despite its larger molecule size.

Tea tree essential oil (*Melaleuca alternifolia***):** Extracted from the leaves of a tree native to Australia, the essential oil contains antibacterial, antifungal, and antiviral compounds, making it popular for natural deodorants and products combating blemishes, athlete's foot, nail fungus, and dandruff. Several studies support its ability to kill viruses, making it beneficial in natural hand sanitizers.

Tea tree hydrosol (*Melaleuca alternifolia***):** The hydrosol reduces the appearance of breakouts and helps keep them at bay, visibly reduces redness and inflammation, minimizes pore size, reduces excessive oil, and visibly tightens skin. It contains the same properties as the essential oil in a less concentrated, less strongly aromatic, and noncaustic form. It can often replace water in formulations to add the benefits of tea tree. It can be used alone, undiluted, as a facial toner or hydrating mist.

TEA-lauryl sulfate: This is a biodegradable detergent and **surfactant** with high foaming capabilities. Research has shown it to be slightly toxic in rats and a significant skin irritant although it is deemed safe for use in cosmetics in lower concentrations. However, often people have sensitivities to detergents and shampoos containing the substance.

Temu kunci (*Boesenbergia pandurata* Roxb.): The rhizome of this Indonesian plant contains **flavonoids** and antifungal, antibacterial, and **antioxidant** properties. Traditionally, it has been used in the treatment of many diseases. Its powerful components have made it popular in antiaging and acne products, plus in foot bombs and nail soaks to treat fungus.

Temulawak extract (*Curcuma xanthorrhiza* Roxb.): Also known as Japanese turmeric, this plant is in the ginger family. The extract is **antioxidant**, antibacterial, and anti-inflammatory. There's some research suggesting it may help lighten skin, however it is mostly used in the treatment of acne and generally found in products such as face creams, cleansers, face oils, and face serums.

Temulawak oil (*Curcuma xanthorrhiza* Roxb.): The oil is a concentrated form of temulawak and has all the attributes of the extract but can be used for different applications. It's used in very small

percentages and normally as spot treatments for acne, blackheads, and pimples.

Thyme cold-pressed oil (*Thymus vulgaris*): Generally infused in another oil, thyme oil is similar to the extract and contains the same benefits in a less caustic form. It has **essential fatty acids** and is used to treat acne, athlete's foot, and skin infections.

Thyme essential oil (*Thymus vulgaris*): This essential oil is one of the strongest **antioxidants** and has been used medicinally since ancient times. It is antifungal, antibacterial, and antiseptic and used to treat acne, infections, fungal infections, eczema, and congested pores. It is also added to hand sanitizers.

Thyme extract (*Thymus vulgaris*): Preliminary research suggests that thyme extract is more effective at killing the bacteria that causes acne than **benzoyl peroxide**, which has led to its inclusion in products for the treatment of acne.

Titanium dioxide: This naturally occurring oxide of titanium is a white fine powder that is used in sunscreens and cosmetics as a colorant; it is also used in soapmaking.

Tolu balsam essential oil (*Balsamum tolutanum*): Made from the resin of the Myroxylon tree native to South America, the essential oil has a lovely warm aroma often used in perfumes and essential oil blends. The blends are added to creams, soaps, shampoos, and face care products. It is often found in massage oils for relieving muscle tension and relaxation. It is also used for eczema, acne, rashes, and infections.

Toluene: This is a solvent and paint thinner that research has shown to be a neurotoxin. It inhibits breathing, may cause developmental damage to a fetus, negatively impacts the immune system, and is potentially linked to blood cancer.

Tomar seed essential oil (*Zanthoxylum armatum*): Made from seeds of a tree native to China and India, the essential oil has a light floral scent that is added to perfumes and essential oil blends. It is an antiseptic, disinfectant, and deodorant used in soaps, hand sanitizers, and facial toners.

Tomato seed oil: This oil is relatively new in cosmetics but is packed with **antioxidants** that can benefit mature skin by alleviating environmental damage. It can enhance and improve skin tone, texture, and softness.

Tribehenin wax: This very soft wax is often combined with harder waxes to achieve the desired texture, viscosity, and firmness in products. It also adds gloss to lip balms, lipsticks, and foundations.

Triclosan: Triclosan is a broad-spectrum antibacterial used in antibacterial soaps, body washes, cosmetics, and toothpaste. Exposure to triclosan can decrease thyroid hormone levels and contribute to forming bacteria-resistant antibiotics. According to the FDA, there's not enough data to assess the level of risk triclosan poses, although ongoing studies, monitored by the FDA, are looking at the potential of skin cancer after long-term exposure.

Trideth-3: This is an **emulsifier** in liquid form as opposed to wax and other semisolid emulsifiers. It is found in many products from floor cleaners and air fresheners to nail polish, face creams, body washes, and lotions. It is considered safe for use in the cosmetics industry, although there is little research on its safety.

Triethanolamine (TEA): Made from a reaction of ammonia with ethylene oxide (a known carcinogen), TEA is a skin irritant for some people and can cause burning, redness, and itching. Much commercial TEA is a combination of 85% TEA and 15% DEA (diethanolamine, which has been linked to some types of cancer). It is used in skin care to balance pH and as an **emulsifier.**

Triisostearyl citrate: A **citric acid** compound that can be derived from a plant or animal source, it is used as a skin conditioner and **emollient.**

Triterpenes: These naturally occur in plants and are one of the most powerful anti-inflammatories as well as being antiviral and antibacterial. They are used in the treatment of cancer and internally to help with insomnia, depression, anxiety, and distraction. Their importance in skin care comes from their profound anti-inflammatory properties, which are key for antiaging, and their antibacterial and antiviral properties for the treatment of acne and psoriasis.

Tuberose essential oil (*Polianthes tuberosa*): The essential oil is very expensive and usually used in high-end perfumes for its floral scent. It is said to ease depression, stress, and anxiety and promote mental clarity.

Tuberose extract (*Polianthes tuberosa*): From a perennial plant related to the agaves, the extract is filled with **polysaccharides** and protects against environmental damage, eliminates pore congestion, resurfaces skin, and prevents dehydration. It also has antiviral and antibacterial properties. It is generally used for mature and dehydrated skin.

Tuberose hydrosol (*Polianthes tuberosa*):
The hydrosol has all the benefits of
the essential oil in a less concentrated
form. It is also a less expensive way to
impart some of the aroma. It can be used
alone as a toner or to replace water in
formulations to increase efficacy and
impart scent.

Tuberose wax (*Polianthes tuberosa*): The
wax is a highly desirable addition to skin
care not only because of its lovely scent
but also for the calming, softening, and
smoothing effect it has on skin. It adds
viscosity, texture, and richness to face
serums and face creams.

Tucuma butter (*Astrocaryum tucuma*):
Extracted from the fruit of a tree native to
Brazil, this is a real butter with no added
ingredients. It is filled with **antioxidants**,
vitamin A, **essential fatty acids**, and
minerals. It protects skin from environmental damage and stress, helps improve
skin elasticity, generates skin cells, and
reduces the appearance of wrinkles. It
provides a profound moisture boost and is
added to body creams, body lotions, and
body butters for antiaging and skin protection. It is also used in lip balms, soaps,
and face creams.

Tulsi essential oil (*Ocimum tenuiflorum*):
Also known as holy basil, tulsi is native to
Asia and highly praised for its medicinal
uses in Ayurvedic medicine. The essential oil calms nerves, protects against
toxins and infections and is antibacterial,
antiviral, anti-inflammatory, analgesic,
and filled with **antioxidants.** While it has
a lot of topical attributes it can be slightly
irritating.

Tulsi extract (*Ocimum tenuiflorum*): The
extract is made from the leaves and
extracted in alcohol, oil, or a solvent. It
is antibacterial, antiviral, and antifungal
and is used to treat acne, athlete's foot,
dandruff, and psoriasis.

Tulsi hydrosol (*Ocimum tenuiflorum*): The
hydrosol has the attributes of the essential oil in a less caustic form and can be
used undiluted to treat acne, aging, congested skin, and for detoxing and in room
and body sprays for headaches, stress,
and anxiety.

Turmeric extract (*Curcuma longa*):
The **antioxidant**, antimicrobial, and
anti-inflammatory properties are
extracted from the root. Most of the
benefits come from curcumin, a powerful
antioxidant that visibly diminishes dark
spots, blemishes, scars, and inflammation.
Turmeric helps soften and smooth skin.
It facilitates wound healing, helps build
and protect collagen, and helps control
psoriasis. Pure curcumin is available for
use in skin care but is not a replacement
for turmeric extract. While the extract
does not have the same concentration as
pure curcumin, it has other benefits and
is often used in conjunction. Additionally,
pure curcumin is highly pigmented and
can discolor products.

Turmeric oil (*Curcuma longa*): Extracted
from the roots, the oil has a beautiful yellow color. Some oils are marketed as pure
but are cut with other carrier oils, so read
the label carefully; pure turmeric oil will
be strongly yellow. While the oil has the
same benefit profile as **turmeric tincture**,
it is much more concentrated.

Turmeric tincture (*Curcuma longa*):
Extracted in different carriers such as
alcohol, **propylene glycol**, **glycerin**, and
vegetable oil, the tincture has the same
beneficial properties as pure **turmeric oil**
but is less potent.

Ucuuba butter (*Virola surinamensis* [*Myristicaceae*]): Extracted from the fruit of an Amazonian tree, this is a pure butter that imparts its golden-brown color to products. The anti-inflammatory and antiseptic properties make it beneficial in the treatment of acne, eczema, and dehydrated skin, and its exceptionally high levels of **essential fatty acids** make it an excellent moisturizer for mature and aging skin. It is used in lotions, body creams, body butters, hard bar lotions, soaps, and face creams.

Valerian root essential oil (*Valeriana officinalis*): Used for its calming, sleep-inducing aroma as well as to help prevent wrinkles and to alleviate eczema, the essential oil is for topical use only, unlike the extract.

Valerian root extract (*Valeriana officinalis*): From a perennial plant native to Europe and Asia traditionally used medicinally as a sedative and sleep aid, valerian root extract is mildly astringent and used in toners and face cleansers. The extract is made through gentle heat extraction and is in alcohol, a chemical solvent, or oil.

Vanilla absolute (*Vanilla planifolia*): While something may be labeled as vanilla essential oil, the delicate aroma compounds in vanilla cannot be separated by water (through steam distillation), which is how an essential oil is generally extracted. Vanilla absolute is made by using a solvent such as **ethanol** to extract the aroma. Vanilla has strong **antioxidant**, antibacterial, and stress-relieving properties. It is also used for psoriasis, depression, and as an aphrodisiac. The absolute is extremely expensive and generally used in small amounts as part of the scent profile of a product.

Vanilla bean extract (*Vanilla planifolia*): The bean extract is made by macerating vanilla beans in alcohol. It has some of the same benefits as the absolute but is less expensive and more readily available. Its dark brown color can discolor products, so it is generally used in small amounts to reduce inflammation and irritation, soothe, calm, protect, and reduce signs of aging.

Vanilla flavor (*Vanilla planifolia*): Vanilla is one of the most popular scents in skin care products, but the absolute is extremely expensive, which leaves the fragrance oil as one of the only alternatives to get the aroma into products. The only issue with the flavor is the carrier. The most common carriers are **propylene glycol** and **canola oil**. The flavor doesn't have any of the beneficial properties of vanilla and is used solely for scent.

Vanilla oil (*Vanilla planifolia*): Vanilla beans are macerated in oil for an extended period to extract both the scent and the nutrient profile. It can replace a non-oil-based extract in oil applications where an **emulsifier** is not used.

Vervain essential oil (*Verbena officinalis*): Extracted from a perennial flowering plant, the essential oil helps decongest pores, clear acne, reduce excess oil, and is an antiseptic and **emollient**.

Vervain extract (*Verbena officinalis*): Vervain extract contains anti-inflammatory and **antioxidant** properties. It alleviates pain, helps prevent tissue damage, and promotes new cell growth. It is used in body creams and salves for joint and muscle aches and pains as well as in skin care products targeting premature aging.

Vetiver essential oil (*Vetiveria zizanioides*): Made from the roots of a perennial grass, the essential oil is expensive and highly regarded for perfume and essential oil blends for skin care body products. It is anti-inflammatory and antiseptic; helps generate new skin cells; accelerates wound healing; relieves muscle pain, nervousness, shock, and insomnia; and is a calming nerve tonic.

Vetiver hydrosol (*Vetiveria zizanioides*): The hydrosol is very rare but highly regarded as it imparts all the attributes of the essential oil and can be used undiluted, which makes it more accessible for face creams and serums.

***Viola hondoensis* W. Becker and H. Boissieu (*Violaceae*):** This is used for its **antioxidant** and anti-inflammatory properties. Studies have shown it to have a positive effect in reducing signs of aging and preventing inflammation, which is one of the causes of skin aging. It inhibits the signs of wrinkles and fine lines while promoting healthy collagen.

Violet absolute (*Viola odorata*): The absolute has all the properties of **violet essential oil** but is extracted through a chemical extraction rather than steam distillation. It is more cost effective and can replace the essential oil in all the same applications.

Violet essential oil (*Viola odorata*): Extracted from the leaves and flowers, the essential oil has the properties and attributes of both. Topically it is good for dry, itchy, irritated, and red skin. It has antiseptic properties and helps visibly reduce pore size. It is an extremely expensive essential oil, making it rarely used or only in small amounts.

Violet flower extract (*Viola odorata*): The flower extract is anti-inflammatory and rich in **antioxidants**, peptides, and salicylic acid (see **beta hydroxy acid**). It is used topically to treat pain and acne, decongest pores, prevent visible signs of aging, and protect skin from environmental stress.

Violet hydrosol (*Viola odorata*): The hydrosol has all the benefits of the essential oil in a less concentrated, noncaustic form that can be used undiluted. It is more cost effective than the essential oil or absolute, making it accessible for imparting the scent and properties to toners targeting acne, face creams, face serums, and body lotions.

Violet leaf extract (*Viola odorata*): The leaf extract can be used alone or in a blend with the flower. It has anti-inflammatory and **antioxidant** properties and is used to promote healthy skin and pores, revitalize skin, and restore luster.

Violet wax (*Viola odorata*): The wax is used for its beautiful aroma and calming, soothing, anti-inflammatory, cleansing, and protecting benefits. It's an **emulsifier** and thickening agent used for viscosity and creamy texture in products ranging from lip balms and hard lotion bars to face serums and creams.

Vitamin A: There are two types of vitamin A, **retinoids** and **carotenoids**. Both convert to **retinol**, which increases new cell production and is generally used in face creams to treat acne and reduce wrinkles. Carotenoids are high in **antioxidants** and prevent damage from UV rays and other environmental stressors and inhibit premature aging. Vitamin A comes in many different forms that differ in strength and how skin recognizes and metabolizes them. All vitamin A causes photosensitivity, so sun avoidance is recommended when using topical vitamin A creams.

Vitamin B3 (niacinamide): Vitamin B3 is common in skin care for its soothing abilities with acne-prone skin, in the treatment of hyperpigmentation, sun-damaged skin, and to reduce fine lines and wrinkles and increase elasticity.

Vitamin B5 (panthenol): This is a common ingredient used in hair care, to help skin retain moisture, as a moisturizer, and to help maintain a protective and conditioning barrier on skin. It is generally not effective enough to be used alone but works in conjunction with other compatible active ingredients.

Vitamin C: One of the most commonly used active ingredients in skin care, this powerful **antioxidant** and anti-inflammatory protects against environmental stressors and visibly reduces signs of aging and damage caused by free radicals. Mature or sun-damaged skin has lower levels of vitamin C, the loss of which is associated with accelerated aging, poor wound healing, and dehydration. Vitamin C also promotes cellular turnover, healthy collagen, production of skin's natural barrier lipids, and skin elasticity and tone. Maintaining healthy levels wards off wrinkles and fine lines while keeping skin healthy. There are many different types of vitamin C, both synthetic and natural.

Vitamin D: Although most vitamin D is synthesized naturally in the body from exposure to the sun, an increasing number of people take internal supplements of this vitamin due to deficiency.

Low levels increase dehydration, eczema, and psoriasis. It is an anti-inflammatory, making it particularly beneficial in the treatment of acne and psoriasis.

Vitamin E: Because vitamin E is soluble in oil, it has extensive transdermal penetration. Studies have shown that vitamin E can help keep both the fluid and moisture content of skin balanced as well as protect skin from environmental stress. Vitamin E is generally combined with other compatible **antioxidants** to make a complete and powerful antioxidant profile that protects skin from signs of damage caused by free radicals. There are different forms of vitamin E, but those generally used in skin care are alpha-tocopherol or tocopherol acetate.

Volcanic ash: This very fine powder is made from the rock and mineral particulates expelled from a volcanic explosion. While harmful when inhaled, the ash is used for its ability to purge and purify, its rich mineral profile, and as a natural **exfoliant**. It is traditionally used in spas to reduce cellulite, blemishes, and wrinkles; relieve eczema and psoriasis; and calm red, irritated skin and rashes. The ash is rich in sulfur, a natural antibacterial often used to treat skin ailments. It is increasingly found in face care products targeting acne or congested pores, and in bath products for cellulite, psoriasis, and detoxification, and in soaps.

Walnut leaf extract (*Nucis juglandis*): This extract is a powerful anti-inflammatory used in bath soaks to reduce swelling and in salves to treat wounds. It is also used for sunburn, itchy skin, rashes, dandruff, and acne.

W

Walnut meat (*Nucis juglandis*): The meat of the walnut is a popular superfood with substantial health benefits. High in **vitamin C**, the meat contains **alpha lipoic acid**, **antioxidants**, anti-inflammatories, and high levels of vitamins and minerals. Topically, for skin care it is finely ground for gentle, nutrient-charged facial **exfoliants**.

Walnut oil (*Nucis juglandis*): Generally cold-pressed from the meat of the walnut, the oil has the same nutrient profile as the meat in a more concentrated form. The oil is also more versatile and primarily used in face oils, creams, and serums, although it has a shorter shelf life, sometimes just 6 to 12 months.

Walnut shell (*Nucis juglandis*): Ground to a fine powder, the outer shell is commonly added to facial cleansers as an **exfoliant**. Walnut shells cannot dissolve in water, so no matter how finely ground they will never be completely spherical, which means the hard, tiny particles can cause microdermabrasions.

Warm adobe clay (illite): Illite clays are a group of minerals with a very similar structure to mica, although they contain more water and less potassium. Each color clay has a slightly different mineral and active component. Illite clays can be confusing as different manufacturers market them using different names. Pay close attention to whether it's an illite and the color, which provides information about which clay it is. Warm adobe clay contains minerals that visibly relieve the appearance of stress by melting muscular tension. The high silicon content in warm adobe clay gives it its firming, toning, and even texture–restoring qualities. It has a high absorption capacity, making it great for congested pores and oily skin.

Water: This is the most common ingredient in skin care, although many natural skin care companies are formulating what they can without water as it reduces the need for preservation systems. Face creams, lotions, cleansers, and other skin and body care products can contain up to 80% water, which makes the water used a powerful component. To increase the efficacy and purity of a product, companies are replacing all or part of the water with hydrosols, coconut water, maple water, or nut milks. There are several types of water besides tap water listed on labels, and since water is such a large percentage of a product, the source of the water is key to the purity of the finished product.

Watermelon extract (*Citrullus lanatus*): Extracted from the pulp and the rind (which contains amino acids) watermelon extract is filled with vitamins and nutrients and has a strong **antioxidant** and anti-inflammatory profile. It has the ability to promote new cell growth and is used in products targeting the effects of aging, sun damage, and dehydration.

Watermelon powder (*Citrullus lanatus*): Made from the pulp, the powder is a concentrated form of all the vitamins and nutrients in watermelon. Powders are becoming more popular in cosmetics as formulating without water eliminates the need for preservatives. Powdered watermelon is used in powdered face masks and **exfoliants** as well as in soapmaking, lotions, and creams.

Watermelon seed oil (*Citrullus lanatus*): Watermelon seeds are first dried to lower their water content, then the oil is extracted through cold process or solvent extraction. The finished oil is filled with **antioxidants**. It is **emollient**, detoxifying, anti-inflammatory, and antiaging. Because it is so stable and has such a long shelf life, it can be used as a carrier oil. It is wonderful for oily skin as it reduces oil production and unclogs pores. It also protects skin against environmental damage and helps expel toxins.

Waxes: Natural and synthetic waxes are used in skin care to seal in and protect hydration, to help form a protective barrier on skin, as an **emollient** and thickening agent, for viscosity and consistency, and to provide stability. They're harder than other types of fats and oils used in products so can enable a product to be semisolid, such as a lip balm or bar lotion, and yet still be hydrating and melt on skin when applied.

Wheat germ oil: Extracted from the germ of the wheat kernel, the oil has a very high **vitamin E** content, **vitamins A** and **D**, amino acids, lecithin, and minerals. It is unstable and has a short shelf life. It is a fairly lightweight oil and when used in skin care products it helps all the ingredients have better transdermal penetration. It is primarily used in high-end face care to prevent, retard, and reverse fine lines, wrinkles, and other signs of aging.

Whey: The liquid part of milk that separates during the cheese making process, whey contains a wide range of quickly absorbed amino acids along with other vital nutrients. Amino acids are the building blocks of healthy collagen. Studies show whey's effectiveness at lightening skin and tackling acne.

White kaolin clay: Also called China clay, this very fine soft powder contains a high level of the mineral kaolinite, which is rich in **silica**. Kaolin clay is one of the gentlest clays and perfect for sensitive and dry skin. Its absorption capacity is lower than most clays, which gives it the ability to soften and mildly exfoliate skin with its gentle particles.

White tea (*Camellia sinensis*): White tea comes from young, minimally processed leaves that contain potent **antioxidants**. It is often used to replace water in formulations to increase efficacy, although the tea and extract are also used together to supercharge the benefits of face creams and serums.

White tea extract (*Camellia sinensis*): The extract comes either powdered or in oil, solvents, or alcohol and is added to anti-aging skin care products.

White willow bark (*Salix alba*): From a deciduous tree native to Europe and Asia, white willow bark's main active ingredient is salicin (an analgesic), but it also contains **antioxidants**. The bark is distilled and made into a tincture or sometimes extracted into a carrier oil or alcohol. Research has shown salicin's efficacy at improving wrinkles and roughness, decreasing pore size, and restoring luster, vibrancy, and firmness when applied topically. It is also anti-inflammatory and antibacterial and is widely used as an acne treatment.

Wild yam extract (*Dioscorea villosa*): Wild yam is filled with **saponins**, which are anti-inflammatory, antibacterial, antiviral, and **antioxidant**. They're also believed to be effective at evening skin pigmentation. The extract is used to improve skin's elasticity; prevent sagging skin; combat hyperpigmentation; soothe and calm irritated, red, and sensitive skin; bring back luster and glow to dull skin, and promote healthy collagen and new collagen production.

Wine: All parts of the grape are used in skin care: leaf extract, seed extract, seed oil, and the skins. Although wine itself is also used, red wine grape peel is primarily used for its **resveratrol** content. There is also wine powder, which is becoming extremely popular in the natural skin care sector as it can be made into powdered masks and **exfoliants** and eliminate the need for preservatives. Wine is also used in soapmaking.

Wintergreen essential oil (*Gaultheria procumbens*): Extracted from the leaves of an evergreen shrub, the essential oil has a high percentage of methyl salicylate, which is related to aspirin and therefore has analgesic properties. It is added to lotions and salves for pain relief, soaps, massage oils, and headache blends. It is also used for scenting soaps and skin care products.

Wintergreen hydrosol (*Gaultheria procumbens*): The hydrosol has all the benefits of the essential oil in a less caustic form and can replace water in formulations to increase efficacy. The hydrosol is used undiluted in body mists to increase energy and vitality and alleviate pain, in facial cleansers to increase circulation, in toners for acne-prone skin, and in lotions for pain relief.

Witch hazel bark (*Hamamelis virginiana*): Native Americans boiled the bark and used it to treat skin ailments. Today it is often used to make tinctures or added to facial toners and cleansers for its mild astringent properties.

Witch hazel hydrosol (*Hamamelis virginiana*): This potent **antioxidant** and natural astringent reduces signs of redness and irritation and makes skin appear tighter, even toned, and more youthful.

Witch hazel leaf (*Hamamelis virginiana*): Clinical studies have shown promising results in the treatment of eczema. The leaf, which can be powdered, dried and cut, or extracted, is increasingly appearing

in lotions, creams, and salves targeting severe dryness, cracked skin, and eczema. It is a powerful anti-inflammatory and antibacterial and has been found to decrease breakouts and be beneficial in treating acne. It is also used for itching, rashes, stings, and insect bites.

***Ximenia Americana* seed oil:** Made by a cold-press process or refined, the oil comes from the seeds of a tree native to Africa. It is used in skin care to help balance oil production and aid lubrication as well as provide softness, suppleness, and hydration to dry skin. It has antiaging and skin cell regeneration benefits.

Yarrow (*Achillea millefolium*): Native to Europe, North America, and Asia, yarrow has anti-inflammatory and **antioxidant** properties. It accelerates wound healing, which, along with its other properties, makes it a powerful ingredient in the treatment of acne. It is also added to toners and cleansers for its mild astringency.

Yarrow essential oil (*Achillea millefolium*): The essential oil is used for acne, wounds, burns, eczema, rashes, scars, and oily skin. It is fairly expensive so when used for its aroma it's generally a small part of a larger scent blend. It is added to skin care products targeting acne, oily skin, and dehydrated skin and added to bath soaks for rashes and eczema.

Yarrow hydrosol (*Achillea millefolium*): The hydrosol has all the properties of the essential oil in a less concentrated form that can be used undiluted or to replace water in formulations to increase efficacy. It is a balancing oil used in toners, cleansers, and face serums to restore, revitalize, and rebalance skin health.

Yellow dock root extract (*Rumex crispus*): From a perennial flowering plant native to Europe and Asia, yellow dock is filled with phytochemicals, potent **antioxidants**, and **flavonoids**. The leaf is also sometimes used although the root has more powerful antioxidant properties. The extract is used in antiaging face creams and serums. It protects skin against environmental damage, maintains healthy collagen, and visibly reduces fine lines and wrinkles.

Yellow kaolin clay: Slightly more absorbent then white clay, yellow kaolin clay is also exfoliating and gentle enough for sensitive skin. It has high levels of titanium, potassium, and silica that together help produce collagen. It is circulation-boosting and used in antiaging and brightening masks and body powders, facial **exfoliants**, and in soaps as a natural colorant.

Ylang-ylang essential oil (*Cananga odorata*): From a tree native to Madagascar, Indonesia, and the Philippines, the essential oil is used aromatherapeutically and in essential oil scent blends to alleviate anxiety, stress, tension, and to lift self-esteem. Topically it can be used on both dry and oily skin.

Ylang-ylang hydrosol (*Cananga odorata*): The hydrosol has all the benefits of the essential oil in a less concentrated form and can be used undiluted or to replace water in formulations to increase efficacy and impart scent. It is used in toners, face cleansers, face creams, and body lotions to treat acne, dermatitis, and eczema,

balance oil production, and for general skin care.

Yogurt: A fermented dairy product, yogurt contains beneficial probiotics that may help with both acne and antiaging. Yogurt is also filled with proteins, the building blocks of healthy collagen. In skin care, full-fat yogurt is used for the benefits the fatty acids provide. It tones and plumps skin and can be used fresh in face care products, body lotions, and soap. Powdered yogurt is also commonly used.

Yuzu essential oil (*Citrus junos*): Made from the fruit peel, the essential oil scent is popular for scenting skin care and bath products. Topically, it's used in skin care products targeting aging and to increase circulation and restore vitality, and in products such as bath soaks and salves to boost immunity.

Yuzu fruit/juice (*Citrus junos*): Often referred to as Japanese grapefruit, yuzu juice, peel, and seeds are traditionally used medicinally. The juice is added to bath products to induce relaxation and relieve pain and in face care products for its high profile of **citric**, **tartaric**, and ascorbic acids. It has the highest level of **vitamin C** of all yuzu components and is said to have one of the highest levels of all citrus. It smoothes skin texture, eliminates dead skin cells, and protects collagen.

Yuzu hydrosol (*Citrus junos*): The hydrosol contains all the benefits of the essential oil in a less caustic form that can be used undiluted or to replace water in a formulation to increase efficacy and impart aroma. Yuzu hydrosol is used for all skin types in everything from face creams to body lotions.

Yuzu peel (*Citrus junos*): A traditional remedy for dry skin in Japan is a soak in the tub with a dozen yuzus floating in it. The active ingredients in the peel infuse the water and help relieve symptoms. The peel contains all the attributes of the essential oil as well as a higher concentration of **bioflavonoids**. It can be used either as an extract or powdered. The powdered peel is used in face masks and facial **exfoliants** geared toward antiaging.

Yuzu seed extract (*Citrus junos*): Used in cosmetics for whitening and smoothing, the seed extract also helps prevent and reverse pigmentation caused by age, hormonal changes, and exposure to UV light by increasing cell turnover, which decreases with age. It also helps build healthy collagen. The extract can be in alcohol, chemical solvent, or in water and **glycerin**.

Yuzu seed oil (*Citrus junos*): Extracted and refined from the seeds, the **antioxidant**-filled seed oil is used to treat dermatitis, excessively dry and dehydrated skin, itchy skin, psoriasis, and eczema.

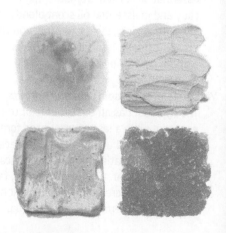

Zinc oxide: Occasionally found in food but more commonly in lotions, makeup, sunscreens, baby powders, athlete's foot products, and other cosmetic industry standards, zinc oxide is used as a colorant, filler, bulking agent, and sunscreen. Non-nanoparticle zinc does not penetrate as profoundly into the skin and is not irritating.

Zinc sulfite: Commonly found as nutritional supplements but also often used in skin care, there is little research to substantiate the claims of its efficacy at treating actinic keratosis lesions, acne, aging, and dandruff. It is astringent and also stabilizes **emulsions**.

4 DIY SKIN CARE Recipes

4

DIY SKIN CARE

Recipes

Our own kitchen cupboards can be a powerful resource for maintaining beautiful, healthy skin. DIY skin care also gives you the opportunity to have complete control over what you put on your skin. However, there are many recipes available that are not only ineffective but also actually create skin issues. For example, many DIY recipes use cornstarch, a natural form of sugar that can grow yeast, which can cause rashes, acne, and diaper rashes. Making skin care products is fun and cost effective, but having reliable sources is key. Just as in the cornstarch example, everything natural is not necessarily good for skin. Remember to always do a patch test when using an ingredient for the first time to ensure you don't have a sensitivity to it.

Ingredients matter! When making your own products, it's always best to use fresh and organic ingredients.

DEEP-CLEAN CLEANSER

45 APPLICATIONS

Clean pores are the gateway to healthy skin. This cleanser will help keep your pores clean so your skin can breathe and function properly.

1 pinch coconut hull or bamboo charcoal
¼ cup finely ground sunflower seeds
2 tablespoons finely ground coconut flakes

Mix all the ingredients in a small bowl. Store in an airtight container. Use within 2 months.

EVERYDAY CLEANSER

45 APPLICATIONS

This mild cleanser is gentle enough for everyday use on even the most sensitive skin. It gently sloughs off dead skin cells, leaving your skin resurfaced, cleansed, and ready to soak up your moisturizer.

¼ cup colloidal oats
2 teaspoons powdered coconut, soy, or goat milk
1 teaspoon almond flour

Mix all the ingredients in a small bowl. Store in an airtight container. Use within 2 months.

PH-BALANCING TONER

60 APPLICATIONS

This toner will wipe away the last traces of dirt and oil your cleanser may have missed. It also primes your pores, protects your skin, and helps keep breakouts away.

2 cups distilled water
1 rooibos tea bag
1 honeybush tea bag
1 teaspoon apple cider vinegar

Combine the water and rooibos and honeybush tea bags in a small pot and simmer until the liquid has reduced to 1 cup. Allow the tea to cool, add the apple cider vinegar, and store in the refrigerator. Use within 2 weeks.

BIOFLAVONOID TONER
(WITH NEROLI)

60 APPLICATIONS

This antioxidant-rich toner will wipe away the last traces of dirt and oil your cleanser may have missed, while preventing visible signs of aging.

2 cups distilled water
1 rose hip tea bag
½ teaspoon citrus peel, including the white part
½ cup neroli hydrosol (optional)

Combine the water, rose hip tea bag, and citrus peel in a small pot and simmer until the liquid has reduced to 1 cup. After cooling, remove the peel (larger pieces work best) and the tea bag. Add the hydrosol (if using) and store in the refrigerator. Use within 2 weeks.

DEEP-CLEANING MASK

MAKES 25 MASKS

An intense pore-purging mask is a key element of a healthy skin care routine. This mask dives deep into your pores, breaks up the dirt and oils, then adheres to them and draws them out so your skin can breathe and function properly.

1 pinch bamboo or coconut hull charcoal
$\frac{1}{2}$ cup kaolin clay
$\frac{1}{2}$ cup French green clay
1 tablespoon distilled water
1 teaspoon apple cider vinegar

1. In a small bowl, mix the charcoal, kaolin clay, and French green clay together and store in an airtight container for up to 1 year.
2. When ready to make a mask, mix together the distilled water and apple cider vinegar in a small bowl.
3. Mix 1 teaspoon of powder with enough vinegar mixture (approximately 1 teaspoon) to make a thin paste.
4. Apply to your face immediately and wear for 5 to 15 minutes. Use within 5 to 7 days.

SKIN-RENEWING MASK

MAKES 1 MASK

This skin-renewing mask replenishes essential fatty acids, vitamins, and nutrients, while dissolving dead skin cells for healthy skin.

$\frac{1}{8}$ teaspoon fresh avocado
$\frac{1}{4}$ teaspoon coconut milk, goat milk, or cow milk yogurt
$\frac{1}{8}$ teaspoon honey or maple syrup
1 small pinch paprika

Place all ingredients in a mini blender and blend or mash by hand to a smooth consistency. Use immediately. Apply to your face immediately and wear for 5 to 15 minutes.

FACIAL SCRUB

16 APPLICATIONS

Gently slough off dead skin cells with this mild facial scrub that is perfect for even the most sensitive skin.

2 teaspoons hemp flour
1 teaspoon finely ground walnuts
1 teaspoon colloidal oats
4 teaspoons honey or maple syrup

Mix all the ingredients together and store in an airtight container in the refrigerator. Use within 2 weeks.

BODY SCRUB

1 APPLICATION

This decadent body scrub is infused with shea butter for ultimate hydration. It's an exfoliator and moisturizer all in one. One tablespoon of scrub is generally enough for a complete application from the neck down.

1 teaspoon avocado oil
1 teaspoon olive oil
1 teaspoon apricot oil
$\frac{1}{2}$ teaspoon shea butter
1 tablespoon sea salt
A few drops your favorite essential oil (optional)

1. In a small bowl, mix together the avocado oil, olive oil, and apricot oil. Melt the shea butter over low heat, add it to the oils, and stir vigorously. Place in the refrigerator.
2. To make the scrub, put the sea salt in a small bowl and saturate it with enough oil mixture to generously coat the salt but not be runny. The type of salt used will determine the amount of oil, as smaller granules will absorb more.
3. Stir in the essential oil (if using).

FACIAL OIL

This combination of noncomedogenic oils is beneficial for all skin types. It will deeply hydrate, balance oil production, and prevent signs of aging. Note: If you have a nut allergy, leave the walnut oil out or replace it with argon oil.

2 tablespoons jojoba oil
2 tablespoons safflower oil
1 tablespoon apricot oil
1 teaspoon rose hip oil
1 teaspoon carrot oil
1 teaspoon walnut oil

1. Mix all the oils in a 1-cup mason jar, close the lid, and shake well. Store the mason jar out of sunlight. Use within 6 to 8 months.
2. After cleansing and toning, place a couple of drops in the palm of your hand, rub your hands together, and massage your face using gentle upward circular motions starting at your neck and moving up.

BODY OR BATH OIL

MAKES ABOUT ³/₄ CUP

This super hydrating oil is rich in essential fatty acids, vitamins, and nutrients that will hydrate you from head to toe.

¼ cup safflower oil
¼ cup olive oil
2 tablespoons avocado oil
2 tablespoons sunflower seed oil
2 tablespoons sesame seed oil (not toasted)

1. Mix all the oils in a 2-cup mason jar, close the lid, and shake well. Store the mason jar out of sunlight. Use within 6 to 8 months.
2. To use as a body oil, apply it in the shower after you've soaped and rinsed, or liberally whenever needed. To use as a bath oil, add 1 teaspoon to 1 tablespoon to bathwater.

REFERENCES

1,2 hexanediol
https://cosmeticsinfo.org/ingredient/12-hexanediol

A

Acacia
https://www. innovareacademics.in/journals/index.php/ijpps/article/view/7901/5978

Acai
https://www.nccih.nih.gov/health/acai/ataglance.htm

Agar agar
https://www.onlinesciencemall.com/blogs/science-blog/what-is-agar

Agave
https://www.britannica.com/plant/Agave

Ajowan
https://www.pharmatutor.org/articles/medicinal-value-of-carom-seeds-overview

Alaea Hawaiian sea salt
https://www.sfsalt.com/alaea-hawaiian-salt

Alfalfa
https://www.healthline.com/nutrition/alfalfa

Allantoin
https://pdfs.semanticscholar.org/170a/99b04fb8a396045846a143941709ed426106.pdf

Almond
https://www.healthline.com/nutrition/almond-oil#section1

Aloe vera
https://www.bcm.edu/news/skin-and-hair/benefits-of-using-aloe-vera

Alpha hydroxy acids
https://www.fda.gov/cosmetics/productsingredients/ingredients/ucm107940.htm

Alpha-lipoic acid
https://my.clevelandclinic.org/health/articles/10980-understanding-the-ingredients
-in-skin-care-products

Aluminum chlorohydrate/chloride
https://pubchem.ncbi.nlm.nih.gov/compound/71586946

Aluminum oxide/alumina
https://pubchem.ncbi.nlm.nih.gov/compound/Alumina

Amaranth
https://www.healthline.com/nutrition/amaranth-health-benefits#section1

Amargo wood extract
https://www.webmd.com/vitamins/ai/ingredientmono-290/quassia

Amazonian lily extract
https://edis.ifas.ufl.edu/pdffiles/FP/FP19800.pdf

Amber extract
http://www.formulatorsampleshop.com/Amber-Extract-p/fss10453.htm

American ginseng
https://www.ncbi.nlm.nih.gov/pubmed/20041778

Ammonium lauryl sulfate
https://pubchem.ncbi.nlm.nih.gov/compound/Ammonium_dodecyl_sulfate

Amyris
https://www.ncbi.nlm.nih.gov/pmc/articles/PMC5435909

Andiroba
https://www.centerchem.com/Products/DownloadFile.aspx?FileID=6970

Aniseed
https://www.sciencedirect.com/science/article/pii/S0308814603000980

Angelica
https://www.ncbi.nlm.nih.gov/pmc/articles/PMC5435909

Anthocyanins
https://www.sciencedirect.com/topics/biochemistry-genetics-and-molecular-biology
/anthocyanins

Antioxidants
https://www.ncbi.nlm.nih.gov/pmc/articles/PMC5514576

Apple
https://www.ncbi.nlm.nih.gov/pmc/articles/PMC5674215

Apple cider vinegar
http://www.pharmaxchange.info/press/2011/03/the-ageing-skin-part-4f-chemical-peels/).

Apricot
https://doctor.ndtv.com/living-healthy/benefits-of-apricot-oil-health-hair-skin-and
-more-1901232

Argan oil
https://www.ncbi.nlm.nih.gov/pmc/articles/PMC5796020

Arnica
https://www.ncbi.nlm.nih.gov/pubmed/15490315

Arrowroot
https://www.sciencedirect.com/topics/biochemistry-genetics-and-molecular- biology
/arrowroot

Asafoetida
https://www.ncbi.nlm.nih.gov/pmc/articles/PMC3459456/

Ascorbyl palmitate
https://pubchem.ncbi.nlm.nih.gov/compound/L-Ascorbyl_6-palmitate#section
=Absorption-Distribution-and-Excretion

Ashwagandha
https://www.researchgate.net/publication/303343480_Studies_of_Ashwagandha_Withania
_somnifera_Dunal

Astragalus
http://www.pnei-it.com/1/upload/bioactive_compounds_from_natural_resources_against
_skin_aging.pdf

Avocado
https://www.ncbi.nlm.nih.gov/pmc/articles/PMC5796020

B

Babassu oil
https://www.ncbi.nlm.nih.gov/pmc/articles/PMC5753019/

Babchi
https://www.sciencedirect.com/topics/pharmacology-toxicology-and-pharmaceutical-science
/psoralea-corylifolia

Balsam of Peru

https://www.ema.europa.eu/documents/herbal-report/draft-assessment-report-myroxy-lon-balsamum-l-harms-var-pereirae-royle-harms-balsamum_en.pdf

Bamboo
https://www.ncbi.nlm.nih.gov/pmc/articles/PMC4659479

Banana
http://www.whfoods.com/genpage.php?tname=foodspice&dbid=7

Baobab
https://www.sciencedirect.com/science/article/pii/S0102695X16300874

Barberry
https://www.ncbi.nlm.nih.gov/pmc/articles/PMC5478785/

Bay
https://www.sciencedirect.com/topics/medicine-and-dentistry/laurus-nobilis

Bee pollen
https://www.thesuperfoods.net/bee-pollen/nutritional-analysis-of-bee-pollen

Beefsteak plant
https://www.ncbi.nlm.nih.gov/pubmed/24898576

Beet sugar
https://www.britannica.com/story/whats-the-difference-between-cane-sugar-and-beet-sugar

Behenic acid
https://academic.oup.com/ajcn/article/73/1/41/4729657

Behentrimonium chloride
https://www.ewg.org/skindeep/ingredient/700657/BEHENTRIMONIUM_CHLORIDE/#
.W6wXcC-ZMnV

Bentonite clay
https://www.universityhealthnews.com/daily/nutrition/3-unexpected-bentonite-clay-benefits

Benzoin
https://www.researchgate.net/publication/230165476_Volatile_constituents_of_benzoin_gums_Siam_and_Sumatra_Part_1

Benzoyl peroxide
https://www.ncbi.nlm.nih.gov/pmc/articles/PMC3088940

Berberine
https://www.webmd.com/vitamins/ai/ingredientmono-1126/berberine

Bergamot
https://www.ncbi.nlm.nih.gov/pmc/articles/PMC5435909

Beta-carotene
https://www.medicalnewstoday.com/articles/252758.php

Beta hydroxy acid
https://pubchem.ncbi.nlm.nih.gov/compound/salicylic_acid

Betel leaf
https://www.science.gov/topicpages/b/betel+leaf+extract

Bilberry
https://www.science.gov/topicpages/v/vaccinium+myrtillus+fruit

Birch
https://www.researchgate.net/publication/297715435_The_medical_importance_of_Betula_alba_-_An_overview

Black cumin
https://www.healthline.com/health/food-nutrition/black-seed-oil-benefits

Black currant
https://www.healthline.com/health/health-benefits-black-currant#side-effects

Black or chebulic myrobalan
http://www.bioline.org.br/pdf?pr16105

Black pepper
https://www.ncbi.nlm.nih.gov/pmc/articles/PMC5600121/#jfds13792-sec-0140title

Black raspberry
https://www.sciencedaily.com/releases/2007/04/070418074348.htm

Black tea
https://www.healthline.com/nutrition/black-tea-benefits#section7

Black willow bark
https://www.onlinelibrary.wiley.com/doi/full/10.1111/j.1468-2494.2011.00645.x

Blackberry
https://www.healthline.com/health/benefits-of-blackberries#takeaway

Blue Cambrian montmorillonite
http://www.rruff.info/doclib/hom/montmorillonite.pdf

Blue lotus
https://www.ncbi.nlm.nih.gov/pmc/articles/PMC4710907

Blue-green algae
https://link.springer.com/chapter/10.1007/978-3-642-66505-9_44

Blueberry seed oil
https://www.ncbi.nlm.nih.gov/pmc/articles/PMC3274736

Bog bilberry
https://www.researchgate.net/publication/263046615_COSMETIC_FORMULATIONS
_CONTAINING_BLUEBERRY_EXTRACTS_VACCINIUM_MYRTILLUS_L

Bolivian rose salt
https://www.seasalt.com/bolivian-rose-salt.html#192=94&202=592

Borage
https://www.ncbi.nlm.nih.gov/pmc/articles/PMC5796020

Boron nitride
https://www.sciencedirect.com/topics/chemistry/boron-nitride

Boysenberry
https://www.ncbi.nlm.nih.gov/pubmed/15686403

Brazil nut
https://www.healthline.com/health/food-nutrition/brazil-nut-benefits#1

Broccoli seed oil
https://www.ncbi.nlm.nih.gov/pmc/articles/PMC4481082

Bromelain
https://www.mdedge.com/dermatology/article/7813/wounds/bromelain-pineapple-extract

Buriti
http://www.ufrgs.br/sbctars-eventos/xxvcbcta/anais/files/1281.pdf

Butylated hydroxytoluene
https://www.ncbi.nlm.nih.gov/pubmed/12396675

Butylparaben
https://pubchem.ncbi.nlm.nih.gov/compound/Butyl_4-hydroxybenzoate

C

C12-18 acid triglyceride
https://www.cir-safety.org/sites/default/files/trygly122017FAR.pdf

Cabbage leaf extract
https://www.ncbi.nlm.nih.gov/pmc/articles/PMC3931201

Caffeine
https://www.healthline.com/health/coffee-benefits-for-skin

Cajeput essential oil
https://wwwlib.teiep.gr/images/stories/acta/Acta%20680/680_8.pdf

Calcium bentonite
https://www.healthline.com/health/calcium-bentonite-clay#2

Calendula
http://www.pnei-it.com/1/upload/bioactive_compounds_from_natural_resources_against
_skin_aging.pdf

California poppy
http://www.dermaviduals.com/english/publications/special-actives/alkaloids
-in-cosmetic-applications.html

Camellia
https://www.dermalinstitute.com/us/news/tag/camellia-japonica/

Camphor
https://www.ncbi.nlm.nih.gov/pmc/articles/PMC5435909/

Canola oil
https://www.ncbi.nlm.nih.gov/pmc/articles/PMC3746113/

Capryl caprylate/caprate
https://www.cir-safety.org/sites/default/files/alkyle032013rep.pdf

Capsaicin
https://www.health.harvard.edu/pain/how-does-hot-pepper-cream-work-to-relieve-pain

Caraway
https://www.ncbi.nlm.nih.gov/pmc/articles/PMC3210012/

Carotenoid
https://www.sciencedirect.com/topics/agricultural-and-biological-sciences/carotenoid

Carrageenan
https://www.sciencedirect.com/topics/food-science/carrageenans

Carrot
https://www.ncbi.nlm.nih.gov/pmc/articles/PMC5435909/

Castor oil
https://www.healthline.com/nutrition/castor-oil

Catnip
https://www.mountainroseherbs.com/products/catnip/profile

Cayenne
http://www.dermaviduals.com/english/publications/special-actives/alkaloids-in-cosmetic-applications.html

CBD
https://www.medicalnewstoday.com/articles/317221.php

Cedarwood
https://www.ncbi.nlm.nih.gov/pmc/articles/PMC5435909

Celery
https://www.ncbi.nlm.nih.gov/pmc/articles/PMC5435909

Cellulose acetate microbeads/cellulose acetate
https://www.sciencedirect.com/topics/agricultural-and-biological-sciences/cellulose-acetate

Ceteareth-20
https://www.cir-safety.org/sites/default/files/PEG-PPG%20Ethers_DR.pdf

Ceteareth-25
https://www.cir-safety.org/sites/default/files/PEG-PPG_ethers.pdf

Cetearyl alcohol
https://www.ewg.org/skindeep/ingredient/701236/CETEARYL_ALCOHOL/#.W66Hdi-ZMnU

Cetyl dimethicone
https://www.ncbi.nlm.nih.gov/pubmed/14555417

Cetyl esters/cetyl palmitate
http://journals.sagepub.com/doi/10.1177/109158189701600107

Cetyl hydroxyethylcellulose
https://pdfs.semanticscholar.org/d664/a7f23cf41aab0d464b7b15071a508280a91a.pdf

Chamomile (German)
http://www.practicaldermatology.com/2010/10/applications-of-popular-botanical-ingredients-in-otc-skincare/

Chardonnay grape seed
https://www.ncbi.nlm.nih.gov/pmc/articles/PMC5052182/

Chaulmoogra oil
https://www.webmd.com/vitamins/ai/ingredientmono-621/chaulmoogra

Cherry blossom extract
https://www.ncbi.nlm.nih.gov/pubmed/25065693

Chia seed
https://www.dermalinstitute.com/us/news/tag/tamanu-oil/

Chinese ash
http://www.pnei-it.com/1/upload/bioactive_compounds_from_natural_resources_against_skin_aging.pdf

Chinese licorice
https://www.tandfonline.com/doi/full/10.1080/13880209.2016.1225775

Chironji
https://www.researchgate.net/publication/282954557_Buchanania_lanzan_spreng_A_veritable_storehouse_of_phytomedicines

Chlorella
http://www.codif-recherche-et-nature.com/wp-content/uploads/2016/02/DERMOCHLORELLA-ZOOM-PUBLICATION.pdf

Chloroxylenol
https://www.researchgate.net/publication/232053156_A_Review_of_Available_Toxicity_Data_on_the_Topical_Antimicrobial_Chloroxylenol

Chromium hydroxide green
https://www.pubchem.ncbi.nlm.nih.gov/compound/22504267#section=Wikipedia

Chromium oxide greens/chromium III oxide
https://toxnet.nlm.nih.gov/cgi-bin/sis/search/a?dbs+hsdb:@term+@DOCNO+1619

Chrysanthemum
https://www.healthline.com/health/food-nutrition/how-chrysanthemum-tea-benefits-health

Cinnamon
https://www.ncbi.nlm.nih.gov/pmc/articles/PMC3854496/

Citric acid
https://www.ncbi.nlm.nih.gov/pmc/articles/PMC3362829/

Citronella
https://www.ncbi.nlm.nih.gov/pmc/articles/PMC5435909/

Clary sage
https://www.sciencedirect.com/science/article/pii/S2221169115001033

Clove
https://www.ncbi.nlm.nih.gov/pmc/articles/PMC5435909/

Cocamide DEA
https://journals.sagepub.com/doi/10.1177/109158189901800204

Cocamidopropyl betaine
https://www.ncbi.nlm.nih.gov/pubmed/18627690

Cocoa
https://www.healthline.com/health/cocoa-butter-for-face

Cocodimonium hydroxypropyl hydrolyzed rice protein
http://www.cir-safety.org/sites/default/files/kerati092015slr%20.pdf

Coconut
https://healthyeating.sfgate.com/benefits-pure-coldpressed-coconut-oil-7169.html

Coenzyme 10
https://www.jaad.org/article/S0190-9622(03)03634-X/fulltext

Coffee
http://www.dermaviduals.com/english/publications/special-actives/alkaloids-in
-cosmetic-applications.html

Collagen protein
https://www.healthline.com/health/collagen-powder-benefits#top-benefits

Colloidal oats
https://jddonline.com/articles/dermatology/S1545961616P0684X/1

Colloidal silver
https://www.mayoclinic.org/healthy-lifestyle/consumer-health/expert-answers
/colloidal-silver/faq-20058061

Comfrey
https://www.ncbi.nlm.nih.gov/pmc/articles/PMC3834722/

Copal
https://www.ncbi.nlm.nih.gov/pmc/articles/PMC5435909/

Copper peptide
https://my.clevelandclinic.org/health/articles/10980-understanding-the-ingre-
dients-in-skin-care-products

Coriander
https://www.ncbi.nlm.nih.gov/pmc/articles/PMC4152784/

Corn silk
https://www.ncbi.nlm.nih.gov/pubmed/24595276

Cornstarch
https://pubchem.ncbi.nlm.nih.gov/compound/24836924

Cornflower
https://www.researchgate.net/publication/313698266_THE_PHARMACOLOGICAL
_IMPORTANCE_OF_CENTAUREA_CYANUS_-A_REVIEW

Cottonseed
https://www.ncbi.nlm.nih.gov/pubmed/11558638

Cranberry
https://www.gundrymd.com/cranberry-seed-oil-skincare/

Cubeb
https://www.tandfonline.com/doi/abs/10.1080/10412905.2007.9699217

Cucumber
https://www.researchgate.net/publication/260228305_Exploring_cucumber_extract_for_skin
_rejuvenation

Cupuaçu
https://www.ncbi.nlm.nih.gov/pmc/articles/PMC4495740

Curculigo (black musli)
http://www.pnei-it.com/1/upload/bioactive_compounds_from_natural_resources_against
_skin_aging.pdf

Curcumin
https://www.ncbi.nlm.nih.gov/pubmed/12676044

Curry
http://www.codif-recherche-et-nature.com/wp-content/uploads/2016/02
/AREAUMAT-PERPERTUA-FICHE-BOTANIQUE-GB.pdf

Cyclopentasiloxane
https://www.osha.europa.eu/en/legislation/directives/regulation-ec-no-1907-2006-of-the
-european-parliament-and-of-the-council

Cypress
https://bmccomplementalternmed.biomedcentral.com/articles/10.1186/1472-6882-14-179

D

D&C colors
https://www.fda.gov/forindustry/coloradditives/coloradditiveinventories/ucm106626.htm

Dandelion
https://www.healthline.com/nutrition/dandelion-benefits#section2

Dates
https://www.healthline.com/nutrition/benefits-of-dates

DEA oleth-10 phosphate
https://www.ewg.org/skindeep/ingredient/701868/DEA-OLETH-10_PHOSPHATE/

Dead Sea clay
https://www.californiaskininstitute.com/treating-body-acne/?gclid
=EAIaIQobChMIm6vswrDb3QIVhWF-Ch3oAw5_EAAYAiAAEgJMD_D_BwE

Dead Sea salt
https://www.sfsalt.com/dead-sea-salt-research

Decyl glucoside
https://www.ncbi.nlm.nih.gov/pubmed/24174472

Decyl oleate
https://journals.sagepub.com/doi/abs/10.1177/1091581803022S106

Deep sea mud/clay
https://www.ncbi.nlm.nih.gov/pubmed/25351016

Dehydroacetic acid
https://journals.sagepub.com/doi/abs/10.3109/10915818509078671

Dehydroepiandrosterone
https://www.ncbi.nlm.nih.gov/pubmed/18242894

Delphinindin
https://www.sciencedirect.com/science/article/pii/S0022202X15331006

Denatured alcohol
https://www.fda.gov/cosmetics/labeling/claims/ucm2005201.htm

Devil's Claw
https://www.uofmhealth.org/health-library/hn-2079001

Dextran
http://citeseerx.ist.psu.edu/viewdoc/download?doi=10.1.1.185.3954&rep=rep1&type=pdf

Dhupu butter
http://www.tropical.theferns.info/viewtropical.php?id=Vateria+indica

Diatomaceous earth
https://www.healthline.com/nutrition/what-is-diatomaceous-earth#safety

Diazolidinyl urea
https://www.contactdermatitisinstitute.com/pdfs/allergens/Diazolidinyl%20urea%20
(Germall%C2%AE%20II).pdf

Dibutylphthalate
https://www.fda.gov/cosmetics/productsingredients/ingredients/ucm128250.htm

Dicaprylyl carbonate
https://www.cir-safety.org/sites/default/files/dialkyl%20carbonates.pdf

Diethanolamine
https://www.toxnet.nlm.nih.gov/cgi-bin/sis/search/a?dbs+hsdb:@term+@DOCNO+924

Diheptyl succinate
https://pubchem.ncbi.nlm.nih.gov/compound/Diheptyl_succinate

Diisostearoyl trimethylolpropane siloxy silicate
https://hpd.nlm.nih.gov/cgi-bin/household/brands?tbl=chem&id=3034

Diisostearyl dimer dilinoleate
https://www.ncbi.nlm.nih.gov/pubmed/14555419

Dill
https://www.mdedge.com/edermatologynews/article/56200/aesthetic-dermatology/dill

Dimethicone
http://www.ewg.org/skindeep/ingredient.php?ingred06=702011&refurl=/product.php#
.W6jxAFJRfMU

Dipotassium phosphate
https://www.ncbi.nlm.nih.gov/pmc/articles/PMC3278747/

Disodium EDTA
https://toxnet.nlm.nih.gov/cgi-bin/sis/search/a?dbs+hsdb:@term+@DOCNO+8013

Disodium laureth sulfosuccinate
http://www.cir-safety.org/sites/default/files/kerati092015slr%20.pdf

DMAE
https://www.ncbi.nlm.nih.gov/pubmed/15675889

DMDM hydantoin
https://www.unilever.com/about/innovation/Our-products-and-ingredients/Your
-ingredient-questions-answered/Formaldehyde-donors.html

Dragonfruit
https://www.sciencedirect.com/science/article/pii/S0308814608011783

Dulse
https://www.ncbi.nlm.nih.gov/pubmed/15833383

Dyer's broom extract
https://www.researchgate.net/publication/264164671_The_production_of_isoflavonoids_in
_Genista_tinctoria_L_cell_suspension_culture_after_abiotic_stressors_treatment

E

Egg
https://www.thedermreview.com/egg-white-mask/

Elastin protein
https://www.elastagen.com/media/The_Science_of_Elastin.pdf

Elderberry
https://www.sciencedaily.com/releases/2007/07/070703172020.htm

Elemi
https://www.ncbi.nlm.nih.gov/pmc/articles/PMC5435909/

Eleuthero
https://www.ncbi.nlm.nih.gov/pmc/articles/PMC5098108/

Emu oil
https://www.medicalnewstoday.com/articles/315535.php

Eperua falcata
https://www.researchgate.net/publication/236644564_Extractives_of_the_tropical_wood
_wallaba_Eperua_falcata_Aubl_as_natural_anti-swelling_agents

Epigallocatechin gallate
https://www.ncbi.nlm.nih.gov/pmc/articles/PMC5796122

Epsom salt
https://www.epsomsaltcouncil.org/uses-benefits/beauty/

Essential fatty acids
https://lpi.oregonstate.edu/mic/health-disease/skin-health/essential-fatty-acids

Essential oil
https://www.takingcharge.csh.umn.edu/explore-healing-practices/aromatherapy/what-does-research-say-about-essential-oils

Ester-C
https://www.ncbi.nlm.nih.gov/pmc/articles/PMC5579659/

Ethanol
https://www.ncbi.nlm.nih.gov/pmc/articles/PMC2596158/

Ethoxydiglycol
http://www.beauty-review.nl/wp-content/uploads/2014/04/Final-report-on-the-safety-assessment-of-butylene-glycol-hexylene-glycol-ethoxydiglycol-and-dipropylene-glycol.pdf

Ethylhexyl olivate
https://www.cir-safety.org/sites/default/files/alkyle_build.pdf

Ethylhexyl palmitate
https://journals.sagepub.com/doi/10.3109/10915818209013145

Ethylhexylglycerin
http://ijpsr.com/bft-article/characterization-and-quantification-of-ethylhexylglycerin/?view=fulltext

Ethylparaben
https://www.ncbi.nlm.nih.gov/pubmed/19101832

Eucalyptus
https://www.ncbi.nlm.nih.gov/pmc/articles/PMC5435909/

Evening primrose
https://www.ncbi.nlm.nih.gov/pubmed/18492193

F

Fennel
https://www.ncbi.nlm.nih.gov/pmc/articles/PMC5435909/

Fenugreek
https://www.ncbi.nlm.nih.gov/pmc/articles/PMC3834722/

Feverfew
http://www.practicaldermatology.com/2010/10/applications-of-popular-botanical-ingredients-in-otc-skincare/

Flavonoids
https://lpi.oregonstate.edu/mic/health-disease/skin-health/flavonoids

Flaxseed
https://www.ncbi.nlm.nih.gov/pmc/articles/PMC3834722/

Formaldehyde
https://www.cancer.gov/about-cancer/causes-prevention/risk/substances/formaldehyde
/formaldehyde-fact-sheet

Frangipani
https://onlinelibrary.wiley.com/doi/full/10.1111/j.1541-4337.2011.00169.x

Frankincense
https://www.ncbi.nlm.nih.gov/pmc/articles/PMC5435909/

French green clay
https://www.ncbi.nlm.nih.gov/pmc/articles/PMC2600539/

G

Gamma linolenic acid
https://www.link.springer.com/article/10.1007/BF03360571

Garlic
https://www.ncbi.nlm.nih.gov/pmc/articles/PMC4734812/

Geranium
https://www.sciencedirect.com/science/article/pii/S2221169115001033

Ginger
https://www.ncbi.nlm.nih.gov/books/NBK92775/

Gingko
https://www.ncbi.nlm.nih.gov/pubmed/15549661

Glacier clay
http://www.clays.org/journal/archive/volume%2023/23-2-153.pdf

Glucose oxidase
https://www.globalhealingcenter.com/natural-health/glucose-oxidase/

Glutamine
https://www.uofmhealth.org/health-library/hn-2856003

Glutathione
https://www.ncbi.nlm.nih.gov/pmc/articles/PMC4207440/

Glycereth-6 laurate
https://www.pubchem.ncbi.nlm.nih.gov/compound/121596024

Glycereth-26
https://www.ncbi.nlm.nih.gov/pmc/articles/PMC4505343/

Glycerin
https://www.ncbi.nlm.nih.gov/pmc/articles/PMC4885180/

Glycerol monostearate (GMS)
https://www.cir-safety.org/sites/default/files/glyest092015TAR.pdf

Glycerol triacetate
https://www.sciencedirect.com/topics/biochemistry-genetics-and-molecular-biology/triacetin

Glyceryl behenate
https://www.accessdata.fda.gov/scripts/cdrh/cfdocs/cfcfr/CFRSearch.cfm?fr=184.1328

Glyceryl cocoate
https://www.ncbi.nlm.nih.gov/pubmed/15513825

Glyceryl dibehenate/distearate
https://journals.sagepub.com/doi/abs/10.1080/10915810701663143

Glyceryl esters
https://www.cir-safety.org/sites/default/files/monoglyceryl%20monoesters.pdf

Glyceryl myristate
http://www.beauty-review.nl/wp-content/uploads/2014/05/Final-report-on
-the-safety-assessment-of-myristyl-myristate-and-isopropyl-myristate.pdf

Glyceryl oleate
http://www.beauty-review.nl/wp-content/uploads/2014/07/Final-Report-on-the-Safety
-Assessment-of-Glyceryl-Oleate.pdf

Glyceryl palmitate
https://pubchem.ncbi.nlm.nih.gov/compound/palmitic_acid#section=Top

Glycine soja
https://www.ncbi.nlm.nih.gov/pmc/articles/PMC5796020/

Glycolic acid
https://www.ncbi.nlm.nih.gov/pmc/articles/PMC4277239/

Glycolipids
https://www.ncbi.nlm.nih.gov/pubmed/22790172

Glycyrrhetinic acid
https://www.sciencedirect.com/topics/neuroscience/glycyrrhetinic-acid

Goat milk
https://drinc.ucdavis.edu/goat-dairy-foods/dairy-goat-milk-composition

Goji berry
https://www.researchgate.net/publication/283675901_Dermatologic_Uses_and_Effects_of_Lycium_Barbarum

Goldenseal
https://www.sciencedirect.com/topics/medicine-and-dentistry/goldenseal

Gooseberry
https://www.researchgate.net/publication/200022975_Anticandidal_effect_of_berry_juices_and_extracts_from_Ribes_species

Gotu kola
https://www.ncbi.nlm.nih.gov/pmc/articles/PMC3834700/

Grape
https://www.mdpi.com/2079-9284/2/3/259/htm

Grapefruit
https://www.sciencebasedmedicine.org/not-natural-not-safe-grapefruit-seed-extract/

Green tea
https://www.ncbi.nlm.nih.gov/books/NBK299060/

Grey salt
https://www.sfsalt.com/french-grey-salt

Guaiacwood
https://www.ncbi.nlm.nih.gov/pmc/articles/PMC5435909/

Guar gum
https://www.sciencedirect.com/topics/agricultural-and-biological-sciences/guar-gum

Guarana
https://www.ncbi.nlm.nih.gov/pubmed/22151935

Guava
https://www.onlinelibrary.wiley.com/doi/abs/10.1111/exd.13151

H

Hawthorn berry
http://pennstatehershey.adam.com/content.aspx?productId=107&pid=33&gid=000256

Hazelnut
https://www.healthline.com/health/beauty-skin-care/hazelnut-oil-for-skin

Hectorite
https://www.sciencedirect.com/topics/earth-and-planetary-sciences/hectorite

Hemp
https://www.healthline.com/health/hemp-oil-for-skin#side-effects-and-risks

Hexanoyl dipeptide-3 norleucine acetate
https://patents.google.com/patent/US6126939A/en

Hexyl laurate
https://www.cir-safety.org/sites/default/files/alkylesters_blue_092012.pdf

Hexyldecanol
https://www.ncbi.nlm.nih.gov/pubmed/23786619

Hexylene glycol
https://doi.org/10.1111/j.1600-0536.1989.tb04728.x

Hibiscus
https://www.dermatocare.com/blog/hibiscus-skin-benefits--exfoliation-anti-aging
-and-hair-growth

Himalayan salt
https://www.medicalnewstoday.com/articles/315081.php

Homosalate
https://www.ncbi.nlm.nih.gov/pubmed/15020197

Honey
https://www.ncbi.nlm.nih.gov/pmc/articles/PMC5661189/

Honeybush
https://www.researchgate.net/publication/273083376_Fact_Sheet_on_Honeybush_Tea

Honeysuckle
https://www.ncbi.nlm.nih.gov/pmc/articles/PMC3577469/

Hops
https://www.onlinelibrary.wiley.com/doi/full/10.1111/1541-4337.12201

Horse chestnut
https://www.centerchem.com/Products/horse-chestnut-extract-hgl-ms-code-40540/

Horsetail
https://www.ncbi.nlm.nih.gov/pmc/articles/PMC4132922/

Hyaluronic acid
https://www.ncbi.nlm.nih.gov/pmc/articles/PMC3970829/

Hydrogen peroxide
https://academic.oup.com/bja/article/118/6/958/3860400

Hydrogenated coco-glycerides
https://www.cir-safety.org/sites/default/files/115_buff3e_suppl.pdf

Hydrogenated didecene
https://www.ewg.org/skindeep/ingredient/702924/HYDROGENATED_DIDECENE/

Hydrogenated lecithin
https://www.ncbi.nlm.nih.gov/pubmed/11358109

Hydrogenated olive
https://www.ncbi.nlm.nih.gov/pubmed/22995032

Hydrogenated polyisobutene
https://www.ncbi.nlm.nih.gov/pubmed/19101833

Hydrogenated soybean
https://www.sciencedirect.com/topics/agricultural-and-biological-sciences/soybean-oil

Hydrogenated starch hydrolysate
https://www.cir-safety.org/sites/default/files/polysaccharide_gums.pdf

Hydrogenated vegetable glycerides citrate
https://www.cir-safety.org/sites/default/files/PEGalk062014SLR.pdf

Hydrolyzed algae extract
https://www.mdpi.com/2079-9284/5/1/2/pdf

Hydrolyzed lupine protein
http://www.cir-safety.org/sites/default/files/pltpep092016slr.pdf

Hydroquinine
https://my.clevelandclinic.org/health/articles/10980-understanding-the
-ingredients-in-skin-care-products

Hydrosols
Catty, Suzanne. *Hydrosols: The Next Aromatherapy*. New York, NY: Healing Arts Press, 2001.

Hydroxyethyl acrylate/sodium acryloyldimethyl taurate copolymer
http://www.cir-safety.org/sites/default/files/ACTAPY122015rep.pdf

Hydroxyethyl urea
https://www.cir-safety.org/sites/default/files/hyurea062018SLR.pdf

Hydroxyethylcellulose
http://www.beauty-review.nl/wp-content/uploads/2014/08/Final-report-on-the
-safety-assessment-of-hydroxyethylcellulose-hydroxypropylcellulose-methylcellulose
-hydroxypropyl-methylcellulose-and-cellulose-gum.pdf

Hydroxyethylpiperazine ethane sulfonic acid
https://books.google.com/books?id=3tfKBQAAQBAJ&pg=PA107&lpg=PA107&dq=HEPES
+topical+study&source=bl&ots=MiSMlR0b91&sig=b8tyWR_cvMjE9-

Hydroxypropyl cyclodextrin
https://www.jpharmsci.org/article/S0022-3549(16)41410-3/pdf

Hydroxypropyl starch phosphate
https://efsa.onlinelibrary.wiley.com/doi/pdf/10.2903/j.efsa.2017.4911

Hyssop
https://www.webmd.com/vitamins/ai/ingredientmono-258/hyssop

I

Illipe butter
https://www.onlinelibrary.wiley.com/doi/abs/10.1002/jsfa.2740600104

Imidazolidinyl urea
https://www.ntp.niehs.nih.gov/ntp/htdocs/chem_background/exsumpdf/imidazolidinylurea
_508.pdf

Indian barberry
http://www.phytopharmajournal.com/Vol6_Issue1_08.pdf

Indian gooseberry
https://www.lifeextension.com/Magazine/2010/7/Unleash-Your-Skins-Internal-Defenses
/Page-01

Indigo
https://www.ncbi.nlm.nih.gov/pubmed/28681622

Inositol
https://www.ncbi.nlm.nih.gov/pubmed/15569619

Iodopropynyl butylcarbamate
https://www.cir-safety.org/sites/default/files/butylcarbamate_rr.pdf

Irish moss (carrageenan)
https://www.webmd.com/vitamins/ai/ingredientmono-710/carrageenan

Iron oxides
https://www.ncbi.nlm.nih.gov/pmc/articles/PMC5316225/

Isoamyl cocoate
https://www.researchgate.net/publication/236067552_Immobilised_lipases_in_the_cosmetics_industry

Isoamyl laurate
https://pubchem.ncbi.nlm.nih.gov/compound/Isoamyl_laurate

Isobutyl acetate
https://pubchem.ncbi.nlm.nih.gov/compound/isobutyl_acetate

Isobutylparaben
https://www.fda.gov/cosmetics/productsingredients/ingredients/ucm128042.htm

Isoflavonoids
https://www.sciencedirect.com/topics/chemistry/isoflavonoid

Isohexadecane
https://www.omicsonline.org/moisturizers-for-patients-with-atopic-dermatitis-an-overview-2155-6121.1000143.pdf

Isoleucine
http://clinical-pediatrics-dermatology.imedpub.com/barrier-repair-therapy-in-atopic-eczemaeffects-of-isoleucine-rhamnosoftceramides-and-niacinamide-facial-and-bodycreams-on-clinical.php?aid=8391

Isononyl isononanoate
https://journals.sagepub.com/doi/abs/10.1177/1091581811428980?journalCode=ijtb

Isopropyl lanolate
https://www.the-dermatologist.com/content/lanolin-wool-wax-alcohol-update

Isopropyl myristate
http://www.nononsensecosmethic.org/wp-content/uploads/2013/12/Comedogenicity-and-irritacy-of-commonly-used-ingredients.pdf

Isopropyl palmitate
http://datasheets.scbt.com/sc-250200.pdf

Isopropyl titanium triisostearate
https://www.cir-safety.org/sites/default/files/organo-titanium%20ingredients.pdf

Isostearamide DEA
http://citeseerx.ist.psu.edu/viewdoc/download?doi=10.1.1.919.1112&rep=rep1&type=pdf

J

Jamaican dogwood
https://restorativemedicine.org/wp-content/uploads/2018/01/Piscidia.pdf

Jasmine
https://www.healthline.com/health/jasmine-essential-oil

Jojoba oil/wax
https://www.mdedge.com/edermatologynews/article/17921/aesthetic-dermatology/jojoba

Juniper
https://www.ncbi.nlm.nih.gov/pmc/articles/PMC5435909/

K

Kacip fatimah
http://www.pnei-it.com/1/upload/bioactive_compounds_from_natural_resources
_against_skin_aging.pdf

Kakadu plum
https://www.sciencedirect.com/science/article/pii/S074000201830515X

Kalahari melon
https://www.researchgate.net/publication/318552260_The_topical_efficacy_and_safety
_of_Citrullus_lanatus_seed_oil_A_short-term_clinical_assessment

Kaolin clay
https://www.researchgate.net/publication/318508286_Characterization_and_Short-Term
_clinical_study_of_clay_facial_mask

Kapoor katcheri
https://www.ncbi.nlm.nih.gov/pmc/articles/PMC3530335/

Kefir
https://www.ajas.info/upload/pdf/147.pd

Kelp
http://www.differencebetween.net/science/nature/difference-between-kelp-and-seaweed/

Kiwi
https://www.ncbi.nlm.nih.gov/pubmed/29470689

Kojic acid
https://my.clevelandclinic.org/health/articles/10980-understanding-the-ingre-
dients-in-skin-care-products

Kokum butter
https://www.sciencedirect.com/topics/agricultural-and-biological-sciences/garcinia-indica

Kombucha
https://www.sciencedirect.com/science/article/pii/S1047279718307385

Kukui nut
https://www.futurederm.com/what-does-kukui-oil-do-for-your-skin/

Kundari
http://www.pnei-it.com/1/upload/bioactive_compounds_from_natural_resources_against
_skin_aging.pdf

L

L-ascorbic acid
https://www.my.clevelandclinic.org/health/articles/10980-understanding-the-ingre-
dients-in-skin-care-products

Lactic acid
https://www.ncbi.nlm.nih.gov/pubmed/8784274

Lanolin
https://www.the-dermatologist.com/content/lanolin-wool-wax-alcohol-update

Laureth-4
https://journals.sagepub.com/doi/abs/10.3109/10915818309141999

Laureth-7
https://www.cir-safety.org/sites/default/files/PEGPPG062013tent.pdf

Laureth-23
http://journals.sagepub.com/doi/abs/10.3109/10915818309141999?journalCode=ijta

Lauric acid
https://www.cir-safety.org/sites/default/files/115_draft_steary_suppl3.pdf

Lauroyl lysine
https://www.cir-safety.org/sites/default/files/aaaamd092013tent.pdf

Lauryl alcohol
https://www.ncbi.nlm.nih.gov/pubmed/12429475

Lauryl glucoside
https://www.ncbi.nlm.nih.gov/pubmed/24617572

Lauryl lactate
https://www.ncbi.nlm.nih.gov/pubmed/8784274

Lauryl laurate
http://www.cir-safety.org/sites/default/files/alkyle032013rep.pdf

Lauryl PEG-9 polydimethylsiloxyethyl dimethicone
https://www.cir-safety.org/sites/default/files/ROPSIL_092014%20_Tent.pdf

Lavender
http://www.practicaldermatology.com/2010/10/applications-of-popular-botanical
-ingredients-in-otc-skincare/

Lemon
https://www.ncbi.nlm.nih.gov/pmc/articles/PMC5435909/

Lemon balm
https://www.ncbi.nlm.nih.gov/pmc/articles/PMC5871149/

Lemon verbena
https://www.science.gov/topicpages/l/lemon+verbena+aloysia

Lemongrass
https://www.ncbi.nlm.nih.gov/pmc/articles/PMC3217679/

Licorice root
http://www.practicaldermatology.com/2010/10/applications-of-popular-botanical
-ingredients-in-otc-skincare/

Lime
https://www.medicalnewstoday.com/articles/304448.php

Litsea cubeba
https://www.science.gov/topicpages/l/litsea+cubeba+essential

Luffa
https://pdfs.semanticscholar.org/ac9f/1f8a23b3b64f83173bafce942d307afba3ea.pdf

Lutein
https://www.sciencebasedhealth.com/Webpage.aspx?WebpageId=68

Lychee
https://www.ncbi.nlm.nih.gov/pmc/articles/PMC3976307/

Lycopene
https://www.lifeextension.com/Magazine/2012/9/Topical-Lycopene-Improves-Skin
-Cellular-Function/Page-01

M

Macadamia nut
https://www.researchgate.net/publication/237671502_EVALUATION_OF_BASIC_PROPERTIES_OF
_MACADAMIA_NUT_OIL

Machilus thunbergii bark
http://www.pnei-it.com/1/upload/bioactive_compounds_from_natural_resources_against
_skin_aging.pdf

Madder root
https://www.sciencedirect.com/science/article/pii/S1319610311002687

Magnesium alum silicate
https://foreveryoung.perriconemd.com/alpha-lipoic-acid-cellular-rejuvenator.html

Magnesium ascorbyl phosphate
https://www.ncbi.nlm.nih.gov/pmc/articles/PMC3673383/

Magnesium aspartate
https://www.cir-safety.org/sites/default/files/alkyl_amides_0.pdf

Magnesium carbonate
https://www.cir-safety.org/sites/default/files/carbonate_salts.pdf

Magnesium laureth sulfate
http://nuph.edu.ua/wp-content/uploads/2016/06/8_Asian-Journal-of-Pharmaceutics-
%E2%80%A2-Jan-Mar-2017-Suppl-%E2%80%A2-11-1.pdf

Magnesium oleth sulfate
https://online.personalcarecouncil.org/ctfa-static/online/lists/cir-pdfs/PR533.PDF

Magnesium sulfate
http://www.epsomsaltcouncil.org/wp-content/uploads/2015/10/report_on_absorption
_of_magnesium_sulfate.pdf

Magnolia bark
https://www.cosmeticsandtoiletries.com/formulating/function/active/81720587.html

Malic acid
https://www.healthline.com/health/malic-acid-skin-care#skin-care-science

Malkangni oil
https://www.researchgate.net/figure/Therapeutic-uses-of-the-plant_fig4_264540128

Maltodextrin
https://www.cir-safety.org/sites/default/files/polysaccharide_gums.pdf

Maltooligosyl glucoside
https://www.ncbi.nlm.nih.gov/pubmed/8234920

Mandarin orange
https://www.ncbi.nlm.nih.gov/pmc/articles/PMC4908842/

Mandelic acid
http://www.nucelle.com/pdfs/article.pdf

Mango
https://www.ncbi.nlm.nih.gov/pmc/articles/PMC3249901/

Mangosteen
https://onlinelibrary.wiley.com/doi/abs/10.1046/j.1365-313X.1998.00073.x

Maple
https://www.acs.org/content/acs/en/pressroom/newsreleases/2018/august
/maple-leaf-extract-could-nip-skin-wrinkles-in-the-bud.html

Marionberry
https://www.ncbi.nlm.nih.gov/pubmed/15686403

Maritime pine
https://www.ncbi.nlm.nih.gov/pmc/articles/PMC3203267/

Marjoram
https://www.ncbi.nlm.nih.gov/pmc/articles/PMC5871212/

Marshmallow root
https://www.ncbi.nlm.nih.gov/pmc/articles/PMC3834722/

Marula oil
https://www.sciencedirect.com/science/article/pii/S0254629911001074

Meadowfoam seed oil
https://www.agresearchmag.ars.usda.gov/1997/feb/meadow/

Menthol
https://www.health.harvard.edu/newsletter_article/Rubbing_it_in

Menthoxypropanediol
https://www.ncbi.nlm.nih.gov/pubmed/27862339

Menthyl anthranilate
https://www.sciencedirect.com/science/article/pii/S101060301731434X

Menthyl lactate
http://www.leffingwell.com/download/Leffingwell%20-%20Handbook%20of%20Cosmetic%20
Science%20and%20Technology.pdf

Methicone
https://www.ncbi.nlm.nih.gov/pubmed/1455541

Methyl gluceth-20
https://www.cir-safety.org/sites/default/files/megluc122012tent_faa_final%20for%20
posting2.pdf

Methyl gluceth-20 benzoate
http://www.innospecinc.com/assets/_files/documents/may_08/cm__1210344657
_Finsolv_EMG-20.pdf

Methyl glucose sesquistearate
https://www.cir-safety.org/sites/default/files/megluc062013tent.pdf

Methylchloroisothiazolinone
https://www.ncbi.nlm.nih.gov/pubmed/2562339

Methyldibromo glutaronitrile
https://www.ncbi.nlm.nih.gov/pubmed/15811027

Methylglucoside phosphate
https://www.cir-safety.org/sites/default/files/megluc092013final.pdf

Methylisothiazolinone
https://www.ncbi.nlm.nih.gov/pmc/articles/PMC4056723/

Methylparaben
https://www.ncbi.nlm.nih.gov/pubmed/19101832

Methylpropanediol
http://www.cir-safety.org/sites/default/files/ADIOLS062016rep.pdf

Methylsilanol mannuronate
https://www.dovepress.com/in-vitro-study-of-rrsreg-silisorg-ce-class-iii-medical-device-composed-peer-reviewed-fulltext-article-MDER

Methylsulfonylmethane (MSM)
https://www.ncbi.nlm.nih.gov/pmc/articles/PMC5372953/

Mexican marigold
https://www.researchgate.net/publication/237813994_The_Use_of_Marigold_Therapy_for_Podiatric_Skin_Conditions

Milk
https://www.ajas.info/upload/pdf/147.pdf

Mineral salts
https://www.sfsalt.com/redmond-real-salt

Moringa
https://www.doctorshealthpress.com/general-health-articles/moringa-oil-benefits-for-skin-hair-health-side-effects-uses/

Moroccan chamomile
http://www.circulating-oils-library.com/en/essential-oils/wild-moroccan-chamomile-essential-oil-ormenis-multicaulis

Moroccan red clay
https://www.sciencedirect.com/science/article/pii/S2214509517300153

Motherwort
https://www.uofmhealth.org/health-library/hn-2132004

Mowrah butter
https://www.researchgate.net/publication/236147474_Mowrah_butter_Nature%27s_novel_fat

Mucilage
https://www.sciencedirect.com/topics/agricultural-and-biological-sciences/mucilage

Mung bean
https://www.pdfs.semanticscholar.org/ac9f/1f8a23b3b64f83173bafce942d307afba3ea.pdf

Mungongo oil
https://www.sciencedirect.com/science/article/pii/S0254629911001074

Mushrooms
https://www.miamiherald.com/living/health-fitness/skin-deep/article1947452.html

Muskmelon
https://www.britannica.com/plant/muskmelon

Mustard
https://food.ndtv.com/health/8-incredible-mustard-oil-benefits-that-make-it-so-pop-ular-1631993

Myristic acid
https://www.acs.org/content/acs/en/molecule-of-the-week/archive/m/myristic-acid.html

Myrrh
https://www.sciencedirect.com/topics/pharmacology-toxicology-and
-pharmaceutical-science/myrrh

N

N-acetyl L-tyrosine
https://www.ewg.org/skindeep/ingredient/700091/ACETYL_TYROSINE/

Narcissus
https://www.ncbi.nlm.nih.gov/pmc/articles/PMC2856661/

Neem oil
https://www.healthline.com/health/neem-oil-for-skin

Neopentyl glycol
https://pubchem.ncbi.nlm.nih.gov/compound/Neopentyl_glycol

Neroli
https://www.hydrosolworld.com/2017/the-benefits-of-neroli/

Noni
https://www.nccih.nih.gov/health/noni

Nonoxynols
https://www.cir-safety.org/sites/default/files/nonoxy122015rep.pdf

Nutmeg
https://www.ncbi.nlm.nih.gov/pmc/articles/PMC5222521/

O

Oak bark
https://www.ncbi.nlm.nih.gov/pmc/articles/PMC3834722/

Oak moss
https://www.tandfonline.com/doi/full/10.1080/13880200600713808

Oats
https://www.dermnetnz.org/topics/oatmeal/

Obsidian clay
https://www.ncbi.nlm.nih.gov/pmc/articles/PMC2904249/

Octinoxate
https://www.healthline.com/health/octinoxate#is-it-safe

Octyl palmitate
https://journals.sagepub.com/doi/abs/10.3109/10915818209013145

Octyldodecyl myristate
https://pubchem.ncbi.nlm.nih.gov/compound/19028571

O-cymen-5-ol
https://journals.sagepub.com/doi/abs/10.3109/10915818409010518

Oenocarpus bataua
https://www.ncbi.nlm.nih.gov/pmc/articles/PMC4964390/

Olive oil
https://www.researchgate.net/publication/305755353_Review_Beneficial_Health_Effects_of_Olive_Leaves_Extracts

Orange
https://www.ncbi.nlm.nih.gov/pmc/articles/PMC3824622/

Oregano
https://www.healthline.com/nutrition/9-oregano-oil-benefits-and-uses#section1

Orris root
https://thedermreview.com/root-extracts-skin-care/

Oryzanol
https://www.ncbi.nlm.nih.gov/pmc/articles/PMC3299446/

Oxidoreductase
https://www.sciencedirect.com/topics/medicine-and-dentistry/oxidoreductase

P

Palm oil
http://www.coconutresearchcenter.org/hwnl_4-2.htm

Palmarosa
https://www.ncbi.nlm.nih.gov/pmc/articles/PMC5435909/

Papaya
https://www.dermatocare.com/blog/7-benefits-of-papaya-for-skin--know
-from-dermatologist

Parabens
https://www.fda.gov/cosmetics/productsingredients/ingredients/ucm128042.htm

Parsley
https://www.ncbi.nlm.nih.gov/pmc/articles/PMC5435909/

Passion fruit
https://pubs.acs.org/doi/abs/10.1021/jf203313r

Patchouli
https://www.ncbi.nlm.nih.gov/pmc/articles/PMC3813264/

Pawpaw
https://www.scialert.net/fulltext/?doi=pjn.2016.23.27

Peach
https://www.medicalnewstoday.com/articles/274620.php

Peanut oil
https://www.ncbi.nlm.nih.gov/pmc/articles/PMC5796020/

Pear
https://www.formulatorsampleshop.com/FSS-Pear-Seed-Oil-p/fss16731.htm

Pecan
https://www.healthline.com/nutrition/9-healthy-nuts#section6

PEG compounds
https://www.ncbi.nlm.nih.gov/pmc/articles/PMC4505343/

Peppermint
https://www.sciencedirect.com/science/article/pii/S2221169115001033

Peptides
https://lpi.oregonstate.edu/mic/health-disease/skin-health/peptides

Perilla seed oil
http://www.imedpub.com/articles/study-on-high-value-application-of-perilla-seed-oil
-and-meal.php?aid=22338

Petitgrain
https://www.ncbi.nlm.nih.gov/pmc/articles/PMC5435909/

Petrolatum
https://www.healthline.com/health/beauty-skin-care/petroleum-jelly#qampa-differences

PHA
https://www.ncbi.nlm.nih.gov/pmc/articles/PMC3047947/

Phenoxyethanol
http://www.safecosmetics.org/get-the-facts/chemicals-of-concern/phenoxyethanol/

Phenylalanine
https://www.healthline.com/nutrition/phenylalanine

Phenylpropanol
https://www.toxnet.nlm.nih.gov/cgi-bin/sis/search/a?dbs+hsdb:@term+@DOCNO+8266

Phthalates
https://www.fda.gov/cosmetics/productsingredients/ingredients/ucm128250.htm

Phytic acid
https://www.healthline.com/nutrition/phytic-acid-101#section5

Phytonutrients
https://www.researchgate.net/publication/313892969_Anti-skin_ageing_phytochemicals_in
_cosmetics_An_appraisal

Pine
https://pubs.acs.org/doi/abs/10.1021/jf048948q

Pineapple
https://pdfs.semanticscholar.org/ac9f/1f8a23b3b64f83173bafce942d307afba3ea.pdf

Pink kaolin clay
https://www.researchgate.net/publication/318508286_Characterization_and_Short-Term
_clinical_study_of_clay_facial_mask

Pink lotus
https://www.sciencedirect.com/science/article/pii/S0308814609013120

Pistachio
https://www.ncbi.nlm.nih.gov/pmc/articles/PMC4890834/

Plankton extract
https://www.researchgate.net/publication/286325112_Glimpses_on_cosmetic_applications
_using_marine_red_algae

Plantain
https://www.uofmhealth.org/health-library/hn-2148003

Plum
https://www.ncbi.nlm.nih.gov/pmc/articles/PMC1173711/

Polyethylene
https://www.ncbi.nlm.nih.gov/pubmed/17365139

Polypodium leucotomos
https://www.lifeextension.com/Magazine/2010/7/ Unleash-Your-Skins-Internal-Defenses/Page-01

Polysaccharides
http://www.scielo.br/pdf/bjps/v48n3/a22v48n3.pdf

Polysorbate 20
http://www.ewg.org/skindeep/ingredient/706089/SODIUM_LAURETH_SULFATE/#.W6Z0iVJRfMU

Polysorbate 60
https://www.bibra-information.co.uk/downloads/toxicity-profile-for-polysorbate-60-1989/

Polysorbate 80
https://www.annallergy.org/article/S1081-1206(10)61024-1/references

Pomegranate
https://www.healthline.com/nutrition/12-proven-benefits-of-pomegranate#section2

Poppy seed
https://ndb.nal.usda.gov/ndb/foods/show/02033?fgcd=&manu=&format=&count=&-
max=25&offset=&sort=default&order=asc&qlookup=poppy+seed&ds=&qt=&qp=&qa-
=&qn=&q=&ing=

Poria cocos
https://www.ncbi.nlm.nih.gov/pubmed/24751506

Potassium sorbate
https://www.ncbi.nlm.nih.gov/pubmed/22570031

Pracaxi seed oil
http://www.tropical.theferns.info/viewtropical.php?id=Pentaclethra+macroloba

Prickly pear
https://www.aromaticstudies.com/prickly-pear-seed-oil/

Probiotics
https://www.sciencedirect.com/science/article/pii/S2352647515000155

Propanediol
http://www.duponttateandlyle.com/pdf/C%26T_Skin_Sensitization_Reprint.pdf

Propolis
https://www.healthline.com/health/propolis-an-ancient-healer

Propylene glycol
https://pubchem.ncbi.nlm.nih.gov/compound/1_2-propanediol

Pumice
https://sciencing.com/pumice-used-5449687.html

Pumpkin
https://www.dermalinstitute.com/us/news/2012/10/the-benefits-of-pumpkin-ingredients-on-the-skin/

PVM/MA decadiene crosspolymer
https://www.ncbi.nlm.nih.gov/pmc/articles/PMC3835651/

PVP
https://journals.sagepub.com/doi/abs/10.1177/1091581817716649

R

Raspberry
https://www.ncbi.nlm.nih.gov/pubmed/15686403

Red algae
https://www.semanticscholar.org/paper/UV-A-sunscreen-from-red-algae-for-protection-skin-Daniel-Cornelia/902037132f533eb070373ff027d56d33c637c751

Red clover
http://pennstatehershey.adam.com/content.aspx?productId=107&pid=33&gid=000270

Red currant
https://pubs.acs.org/doi/abs/10.1021/jf902806j

Reishi mushroom
https://www.healthline.com/nutrition/reishi-mushroom-benefits#section1

Resveratrol
https://www.livescience.com/52541-phytonutrients.html

Retinaldehyde
https://www.ncbi.nlm.nih.gov/pmc/articles/PMC2699641/

Retinoids
https://www.cir-safety.org/sites/default/files/Retinol_DAR.pdf

Retinol
https://www.ncbi.nlm.nih.gov/pmc/articles/PMC2699641/

Retinyl palmitate
https://lpi.oregonstate.edu/mic/vitamins/vitamin-A

Rhassoul clay
https://www.ncbi.nlm.nih.gov/pmc/articles/PMC2904249/

Ribwort
https://www.ncbi.nlm.nih.gov/pmc/articles/PMC3834722/

Rice
https://www.webmd.com/vitamins/ai/ingredientmono-852/rice-bran

R-lipoic acid
https://lpi.oregonstate.edu/mic/dietary-factors/lipoic-acid

Rock rose
https://www.ncbi.nlm.nih.gov/pmc/articles/PMC5435909/

Roman chamomile
https://www.sciencedirect.com/topics/agricultural-and-biological-sciences/chamaemelum-nobile

Rooibos
https://www.ncbi.nlm.nih.gov/pmc/articles/PMC3967803/

Rose
https://www.ncbi.nlm.nih.gov/pmc/articles/PMC5796020/

Rose geranium
http://www.acanceresearch.com/cancer-research/pelargonium-graveolens-rose-geranium--a-novel-therapeutic-agent-for-antibacterial-antioxidant-antifungal-and-diabetics.pdf

Rosemary
https://www.medicalnewstoday.com/articles/266370.php

Rosewood
https://www.ncbi.nlm.nih.gov/pmc/articles/PMC5435909/

Royal jelly
https://www.healthline.com/nutrition/royal-jelly#section9

S

Saccharide isomerate
https://www.cir-safety.org/sites/default/files/saccharides.pdf

Saccharomyces lysate
https://www.researchgate.net/publication/26688190_Bifidobacterium_longum_lysate_a_new
_ingredient_for_reactive_skin

Sacha inchi oil
https://www.hindawi.com/journals/ecam/2013/950272/abs/

Safflower seed oil
https://www.ncbi.nlm.nih.gov/pmc/articles/PMC5796020/

Saffron
https://www.ncbi.nlm.nih.gov/pmc/articles/PMC3862060/

Sage
https://www.ncbi.nlm.nih.gov/pubmed/21391115

Sake
https://www.britannica.com/topic/sake

Sal seed
http://www.worldagroforestry.org/treedb2/AFTPDFS/Shorea_robusta.PDF

Saponins
http://www.dermaviduals.com/english/publications/special-actives/saponins-in
-skin-care.html

Savory
https://www.onlinelibrary.wiley.com/doi/abs/10.1002/ejlt.201000547

Saw palmetto
https://www.healthline.com/health/saw-palmetto-hair-loss#side-effects

Schisandra
https://www.cosmeticsandtoiletries.com/formulating/function/active/premium-Narcissus
-Tazetta-and-emSchizandra-Chinensisem-to-Regulate-Youth-Gene-ClustersAn-In-vitro
-Analysis-226957861.html

Sea buckthorn
https://www.researchgate.net/publication/267307083_Sea_Buckthorn_Oil_for_skin_health_and_Beauty_from_Within

Sea salt
https://www.ncbi.nlm.nih.gov/pubmed/15689218

Seaweed
https://www.tandfonline.com/doi/abs/10.1080/10715762.2017.1355550?src=recsys&journalCode=ifra20

Senna alata
https://wwwlib.teiep.gr/images/stories/acta/Acta%20597/597_28.pdf

Sesame
https://www.ncbi.nlm.nih.gov/pmc/articles/PMC5796020/

Sesbania
https://www.hort.purdue.edu/newcrop/duke_energy/Sesbania_grandiflora.html

Shea butter/oil
https://www.ncbi.nlm.nih.gov/pmc/articles/PMC5796020/

Shiitake mushroom
https://www.healthline.com/nutrition/shiitake-mushrooms#section2

Silica
https://www.ncbi.nlm.nih.gov/pmc/articles/PMC4938278/

Silk amino acids
https://www.ncbi.nlm.nih.gov/pmc/articles/PMC4822939/

Skullcap
https://www.dermascope.com/scope-this/skullcap-extract-in-skin-care

Slippery elm
https://www.frostburg.edu/fsu/assets/File/ACES/ulmus%20rubra%20-final.pdf

Sodium benzoate
https://www.ncbi.nlm.nih.gov/pubmed/11766131

Sodium bicarbonate
https://www.jaad.org/article/S0190-9622(09)00493-9/fulltext

Sodium coceth sulfate
https://online.personalcarecouncil.org/ctfa-static/online/lists/cir-pdfs/PR533.PDF

Sodium hydroxide
https://pubchem.ncbi.nlm.nih.gov/compound/sodium_hydroxide

Sodium laureth sulfate
http://www.ewg.org/skindeep/ingredient/706089/SODIUM_LAURETH_SULFATE/#.W6Z0iVJRfMU

Sodium PCA
https://www.cir-safety.org/sites/default/files/pca.pdf

Solar-evaporated Pacific sea salt
https://www.mayoclinic.org/healthy-lifestyle/nutrition-and-healthy-eating/expert-answers/sea-salt/faq-20058512

Sorghum
https://scialert.net/fulltext/?doi=ajft.2007.79.86

Soy
https://www.ncbi.nlm.nih.gov/pmc/articles/PMC5188409/

Spearmint
https://www.medicalnewstoday.com/articles/266128.php

Spirulina
https://www.omicsonline.org/open-access/clinical-efficacy-of-dermocosmetic-formulations-containing-spirulina-extract-on-young-and-mature-skin-effects-on-the-skin-hydrolipidic-barrier-and-structural-properties-2167-065X-1000144.pdf

Squalane
https://www.ncbi.nlm.nih.gov/pmc/articles/PMC4885180/

St. John's wort
https://www.ncbi.nlm.nih.gov/pmc/articles/PMC5411873/

Strawberry
https://www.medicalnewstoday.com/articles/271285.php

Stinging nettle
https://www.ncbi.nlm.nih.gov/pmc/articles/PMC3529973/

Suganda bala
http://www.imedpub.com/articles/antimicrobial-and-antiinflammatoryactivity-of-bioactive-components-ofpavonia-odorata-wild.pdf

Sugar, cane
https://www.ncbi.nlm.nih.gov/pubmed/19245467

Sunflower seed
http://www.practicaldermatology.com/2010/10/applications-of-popular-botanical
-ingredients-in-otc-skincare/

Sunscreen chemicals
https://www.ewg.org/sunscreen/report/the-trouble-with-sunscreen-chemicals/

Sygyzium
https://www.innovareacademics.in/journals/index.php/ijpps/article/view/7901/5978

T

***Tabernaemontana divaricata* Linn.**
https://www.pharmatutor.org/articles/antioxidant-activity-of-flowers-and-leave
s-of-tabernaemontana-divaricata-linn

Table salt
https://www.mayoclinic.org/healthy-lifestyle/nutrition-and-healthy-eating/expert-answers
/sea-salt/faq-20058512

Talcum powder
https://www.fda.gov/cosmetics/productsingredients/ingredients/ucm293184.htm

Tamanu oil
https://www.healthline.com/health/psoriasis/tamanu-oil-psoriasis-healer

Tamarillo
https://pdfs.semanticscholar.org/ac9f/1f8a23b3b64f83173bafce942d307afba3ea.pdf

Tarragon essential oil
https://www.sciencedirect.com/science/article/pii/S0278691512005303

Tartaric acid
https://pubchem.ncbi.nlm.nih.gov/compound/tartaric_acid

Tea tree
http://www.practicaldermatology.com/2010/10/applications-of-popular
-botanical-ingredients-in-otc-skincare/

TEA-lauryl sulfate
https://journals.sagepub.com/doi/10.3109/10915818209021267

Temu kunci
https://www.sciencedirect.com/science/article/pii/S1876619614001922

Temulawak
https://www.ema.europa.eu/documents/herbal-report/final-assessment-report
-curcuma-xanthorrhiza-roxb-c-xanthorrhiza-d-dietrich-rhizoma_en.pdf

Thyme
https://www.jstage.jst.go.jp/article/jos/65/8/65_ess16042/_article

Titanium dioxide
https://www.ncbi.nlm.nih.gov/pmc/articles/PMC2855360/

Tolu balsam
https://www.ema.europa.eu/documents/herbal-report/draft-assessment-report
-myroxylon-balsamum-l-harms-var-pereirae-royle-harms-balsamum_en.pdf

Toluene
http://www.cybra.lodz.pl/Content/10761/PJOM_1990_Vol_3_No_1_(109-116).pdf

Tomar seed essential oil
https://www.sciencedirect.com/science/article/pii/S0378874118318245

Tomato seed oil
https://www.cosmeticsdesign.com/Article/2012/08/08/Botanic-Innovation-targets
-anti-oxidant-rich-tomato-seed-oil-at-hair-and-skin-care

Tribenehin wax
https://pubchem.ncbi.nlm.nih.gov/compound/Tribehenin

Triclosan
https://www.fda.gov/ForConsumers/ConsumerUpdates/ucm205999.htm

Trideth-3
https://hpd.nlm.nih.gov/cgi-bin/household/brands?tbl=chem&id=729

Triethoanolamine
http://www.ewg.org/skindeep/ingredient/706639/TRIETHANOLAMINE/#.W6hGSlJRfMU

Triisostearyl citrate
http://www.alegesanatos.ro/dbimg/files/Citric%20acid.pdf

Triterpenes
https://www.mdedge.com/edermatologynews/article/9403/aesthetic-dermatology
/triterpenoids

Tuberose
https://www.jstage.jst.go.jp/article/sccj1979/30/1/30_1_77/_article/-char/en

Tucuma butter
https://www.hallstar.com/product/tucuma-seed-butter-ultra-ref/

Tulsi
http://www.ijdr.in/article.asp?issn=0970-9290;year=2010;volume=21;issue=3;spage=357;epage=359;aulast=Agarwal

Turmeric
https://www.healthline.com/health/turmeric-for-skin

U

Ucuuba butter
https://www.sciencedirect.com/science/article/pii/S0378874108007253

V

Valerian
https://www.ods.od.nih.gov/factsheets/Valerian-HealthProfessional/

Vanilla
https://pubs.acs.org/doi/abs/10.1021/ja02025a019

Vervain
https://skums.ac.ir/Dorsapax/Data/Sub_39/File/ProfessorsArticles_etoolsfile1_90d3ffc4-72ba-49d4-a5fb-145add444b04p976-c2706f1a-e582-4f9a-9d4a-bbbc84ff3fb4.pdf

Vetiver
http://www.plantsjournal.com/vol1Issue1/Issue_may_2013/6.pdf

Viola hondoensis
http://www.pnei-it.com/1/upload/bioactive_compounds_from_natural_resources_against_skin_aging.pdf

Violet
https://www.centerchem.com/Products/DownloadFile.aspx?FileID=6939

Vitamin A
https://lpi.oregonstate.edu/mic/health-disease/skin-health/vitamin-A

Vitamin B3
http://www.dermatologytimes.com/clinical-pharmacology/topical-vitamins-hold-promise-face-challenges

Vitamin B5
https://www.healthline.com/health/vitamin-watch-what-does-b5-do#daily-intake

Vitamin C
https://lpi.oregonstate.edu/mic/health-disease/skin-health/vitamin-C

Vitamin D
https://lpi.oregonstate.edu/mic/health-disease/skin-health/vitamin-D

Vitamin E
https://www.mdedge.com/edermatologynews/article/111743/aesthetic-dermatology/update-vitamin-e

Volcanic ash
https://www.sciencedaily.com/terms/volcanic_ash.htm

W

Walnut
https://www.ncbi.nlm.nih.gov/pmc/articles/PMC3834722/

Warm adobe clay
https://www.britannica.com/science/illite

Watermelon
https://www.researchgate.net/publication/267935195_Watermelons_and_Health

Wheat germ oil
https://www.pharmanewsonline.com/health-wonders-of-wheat-germ-oil/

Whey
https://www.ajas.info/upload/pdf/147.pdf

White kaolin clay
https://www.webmd.com/vitamins/ai/ingredientmono-44/kaolin

White tea
https://www.healthline.com/nutrition/white-tea-benefits

White willow bark
https://www.ncbi.nlm.nih.gov/pubmed/20883292

Wild yam
https://www.gundrymd.com/wild-yam-extract-skincare/

Wintergreen
https://www.ncbi.nlm.nih.gov/pmc/articles/PMC3995208/

Witch hazel
https://www.ncbi.nlm.nih.gov/pmc/articles/PMC3834722/

X

Ximenia Americana **seed oil**
https://www.sciencedirect.com/science/article/pii/S0254629911001074

Y

Yarrow
https://www.ncbi.nlm.nih.gov/pmc/articles/PMC5435909/

Yellow dock
https://www.ncbi.nlm.nih.gov/pubmed/20623623

Yellow kaolin clay
https://www.durablehealth.net/kaolin-clay/white-red-yellow-pink
-kaolin-clays-benefits-uses/

Ylang-ylang
https://www.ncbi.nlm.nih.gov/pmc/articles/PMC5435909/

Yogurt
https://www.sciencedirect.com/science/article/pii/S2352647515000155

Yuzu
http://www.oryza.co.jp/html/english/pdf/Yuzu_Seed_Extract_ver3.0M.pdf

Z

Zinc oxide
https://www.ncbi.nlm.nih.gov/pmc/articles/PMC4120804/

Zinc sulfite
https://www.academic.oup.com/jn/article/135/5/1102/4663877

INDEX

ACKNOWLEDGMENTS

Writing a book on a combination of topics with the inclusion of 1,000 cosmetic ingredient definitions was a daunting task! But the support and encouragement from my publishing team was invaluable. From Elizabeth, who patiently got the process started, to Nana K., who wrote the most comprehensive outline, to Meredith, who took my disorganized manuscript and polished it. Thank you.

To my fans who make my days brighter. To hear how their skin has changed, how I've empowered them with education to make choices they're comfortable with, allowed them to make effective products at home, and brought joy to their life is an endless source of inspiration.

I thank my family, extended family, and staff for putting up with and supporting me during the writing of this book, and always.

A huge thanks goes to you, the reader, for demanding information to be able to make informed choices about what you put on your body. To be able to provide that information is humbling.

In gratitude and good health,

Deborah

Deborah Burnes has been "at the forefront of the natural beauty product revolution" for at least two decades. Concerned about the rapid proliferation of chemical-laden products, and convinced that nature is the ultimate innovator, Deborah married her knowledge of chemistry, biology, and cosmetology with studies in medicinal herbs, nutrition, and environmental sustainability to launch Sumbody, an extensive range of skin care, body care, and color cosmetics formulated with pure, potent, wholesum natural and organic ingredients.

She has written two other books, *Natural Beauty Skin Care: 110 Organic Formulas for a Radiant You!* and *Look Great, Live Green*. Deborah's products are regularly highlighted on TV and in magazines. Her popular blog is www.Sumbody.com/Blog.